D1626986

The
Shiva Samhita

The

Shiva Samhita

A Critical Edition

and

An English Translation

James Mallinson

YogaVidya.com

An important message to our readers:

The asanas in this book should not be attempted without the supervision of an experienced teacher or prior experience. Many of the other practices should not be attempted at all. The ideas expressed in this book should not be used to diagnose, prescribe, treat, cure, or prevent any disease, illness, or individual health problem. Consult your health care practitioner for individual health care. YogaVidya.com LLC shall not be liable for any direct, indirect, incidental, special, consequential, or punitive damages resulting from the use of this book.

YogaVidya.com, PO Box 569, Woodstock NY 12498-0569 USA

Copyright ©2007 YogaVidya.com LLC. All rights reserved

Read the Originals is a trademark of YogaVidya.com LLC.
YogaVidya.com is a registered trademark of YogaVidya.com LLC.

First edition

∞ The paper used in this book meets the requirements of the American National Standards Institute/National Information Standards Organization Permanence of Paper for Publications and Documents in Libraries and Archives, ANSI/NISO Z39.48-1992.

Manufactured in the United States of America

British Library Cataloguing-in-Publication Data
A catalogue record for this book is available from the British Library.

Library of Congress Cataloging-in-Publication Data
Sivasamhita. English & Sanskrit.
  The Shiva samhita : a critical edition and an English translation / James Mallinson. — 1st ed.
    p. cm.
  Includes index.
  ISBN 978-0-9716466-4-3 (cloth : alk. paper)
  ISBN 978-0-9716466-5-0 (pbk. : alk. paper)
  1. Hatha yoga—Early works to 1800. I. Mallinson, James, 1970– II. Title.
  BL1238.56.H38S58513 2007
  294.5'9—dc22   2006052817

Loretta rocks.

For Claudia and Lily

Contents

Introduction

COMPOSED OVER five centuries ago, the *Shiva Samhita* is one of the most celebrated root texts of Hatha Yoga. It includes beautiful teachings found nowhere else. This edition contains the original Sanskrit, properly edited and printed for the first time, and a new, accurate translation thereof. It also features photographs of the asanas and mudras described therein.

The book is addressed by Shiva to his consort Parvati, and the title means "The Collection [of Verses] of Shiva." It proclaims a Yoga teaching, yet also calls itself a tantra. It is such an eclectic collection of Yogic lore that a thorough breakdown of its contents would be nearly as long as the text itself, but the topics covered in its five chapters can be summarized as follows.

The first chapter starts with the declaration that "there is one eternal true knowledge" and goes on to mention various methods of liberation and philosophical standpoints, all of which can be transcended by the teachings on Yoga found in the *Shiva Samhita*. Most of the rest of the chapter is an exposition of nondual Vedantic philosophy in the style of the southern Tantric school of Sri Vidya.

The second chapter describes the macrocosm's microcosmic equivalents in the body, the nadis or channels, the internal fire, and the workings of the jiva, or vital principle. The third chapter describes the winds in the body, the importance of the guru, the four stages of Yoga, the fivefold elemental visualizations, and four asanas. The fourth chapter details eleven mudras, which are techniques that result in various Yogic attainments and magical powers, in particular the raising of Kundalini.

The fifth chapter is the longest and most diverse. It describes the obstacles to liberation, the four types of aspirants, the magical technique of shadow gazing, the internal sound, esoteric centers and energies in the body including Kundalini and the seven lotuses, "the king of kings of Yogas," and a threefold mantra whose repetition leads, via global domination, to absorption in the Absolute.

The *Shiva Samhita* was cited extensively by such eminent medieval authors as Narayana Tirtha, Shivananda Sarasvati, Ballala, and Bhavadeva Mishra. The latter's *Yuktabhavadeva* was composed in 1623 CE, while Shivananda Sarasvati's *Yoga-cintamani* can be dated to approximately 1600 CE. So, allowing some time for the *Shiva Samhita* to attain a reputation making it worthy of citation, we can suppose 1500 CE as the latest date for the text's composition. The text borrows verses from earlier works, including the *Amritasiddhi* and the *Dattatreya Yoga Shastra*. The latter can be dated to approximately the thirteenth century CE, so we can say that the *Shiva Samhita* was probably composed between 1300 and 1500 CE.

It also contains a good clue as to where it was composed. In the fifth chapter there is a rather forced attempt to impose a new (and topographically unlikely) homology on top of the usual schema in which the Ida and Pingala nadis are equated with the Ganga, or Ganges, and Yamuna rivers, and the central Sushumna nadi with the Sarasvati, the legendary subterranean river said to join the Ganga and Yamuna at their confluence in Prayaga, modern-day Allahabad. In verses 5.132-134 and 5.138-139, the Ganga is instead equated with Sushumna, and Ida and Pingala with the Varana and Asi rivers, small tributaries of the Ganga which flow in Varanasi. Thus it seems likely that the text was composed in or around Varanasi. The author or compiler, however, remains unknown.

The translation of the *Shiva Samhita* into English by Chandra Vasu in 1914 found an audience amongst Yoga aficionados around the globe. It might be asked if another translation is needed. (There have been other translations too, but all are either based on Vasu's or are inferior to his.) Well, there are many shortcomings to Vasu's work; I shall mention only the most important ones here. Firstly, his translation is often inaccurate. Secondly, there is no indication of which Sanskrit manuscript(s) he used, or how he used them. Thirdly, he prudishly omits an important practice, Vajrolimudra, which is found in this volume in verses 4.78-104.

When I undertook this translation, I decided to use the only critical edition of the text available, the one published in 1999 by the Kaivalya Dham Yoga Research Institute. They had painstakingly collated thirteen manuscripts and three printed editions, duly recording several thousand variant readings. However, when I examined their choice of readings, I found that, despite the good intentions they espouse in their introduction, they had not applied the critical rigor necessary for the undertaking. I have thus re-edited the text, checking every single one of the several thousand variant readings. I found it necessary to adopt different readings in over three hundred places. Please consult the YogaVidya.com web site for information about these readings and the reasons for their adoption.

Thus the Sanskrit in this book is the first to be based on a truly critical study of the manuscripts of the text. I wish I could say that this means that the translation is also the first to be truly coherent. Unfortunately this is not so. There are two reasons for this. Firstly, in some places the readings found in all the manuscripts are very corrupt and it is difficult to make sense of them. Secondly, the text is an eclectic collection of Yogic teachings and some of these teachings contradict each other. Neither of these points has been addressed by previous editors and translators of the text. By means of emendation and careful adoption of variant readings, I have managed to make some sense of all the difficult passages, but one or two of them should still be taken with a pinch of salt, for example, the description of Kundalini and her attendant mantras in verses 5.79-83.

Some of the problems caused by the text's composite nature are less problematic. For example, chapter four is devoted to mudras. It starts with a eulogistic description of Yonimudra, culminating in the statement that by Yonimudra the yogi can achieve anything, even liberation. Shiva then gives a list of ten mudras that he is going to teach, the very best mudras, and Yonimudra is not among them. Similarly, in verses 3.35-37 there is a list of obstacles to liberation which are to be avoided by the yogi, and then in verses 5.3-8 there is another list, with only slight overlaps between the two. To cite a third instance, in verse 4.110 the yogi is told to adopt Muktasana, which is not among the four asanas taught in chapter three. These contradictions are trivial and merely serve to indicate that the text is a compilation, like many Hatha Yogic works. However, there is one contradiction that is harder to resolve. In the description of Vajrolimudra, verses 4.92-3 and 4.103 tell how the yogi can be a bhogi, enjoying worldly pleasures while on the path to siddhis, or Yogic powers. Very shortly afterwards, in verse 5.2, we read that bhoga, enjoyment, is the ultimate obstacle to liberation and, in verse 5.11, that drawing milk up the urethra, one of the preliminary practices for perfecting Vajrolimudra, is an obstacle to liberation. Now it may simply be that we are hearing separate instructions for the two traditional types of Tantric aspirant, namely bubhukshus, those desirous of siddhis, and mumukshus, those desirous of liberation, but the unqualified juxtaposition is jarring, particularly in light of the last verses of the text, wherein the householder is said to be able to obtain siddhis and become liberated by means of the techniques of Yoga—and still have fun!

Despite these problems, the *Shiva Samhita* is an important text and a repository of teachings not found elsewhere in the Hatha Yogic canon. Unlike other manuals of Hatha Yoga, it does not teach a six- or eight-limbed Yoga. Its pranayama is strikingly simple, and it only mentions pratyahara and samadhi in passing. Its most systematic and thorough teaching is that on mudras found in chapter four. Complementing this are its many subtle body visualizations and mantra techniques, found for the most part in chapter five. These beautiful meditations often have no parallels in other Hatha Yogic texts, but rather echo Tantric texts of the Sri Vidya tradition in which the siddhi of becoming like the god of love and attracting women is commonplace.

Another feature of the text which sets it apart from most other works on Hatha Yoga is that it makes no mention of the Natha school of yogis, traditionally said to be the originators of Hatha Yoga. Indeed, there is little in the text which explicitly connects it with any specific tradition, apart from three mentions of the goddess Tripura (verses 5.84, 5.240, and 5.252) and the text's philosophical doctrines, which indicate that it is a product of the school of Sri Vidya, which was adopted by the Shaiva Shankaracharyas of Shringeri and Kanchipuram. As Hatha Yoga, originally the preserve of the unorthodox Nathas, grew in popularity in the medieval period, the orthodox Shaivas sought to incorporate it within their soteriology, and thus the *Shiva Samhita* may be an example of this appropriation.

In conclusion, I labored painstakingly for many months to give you a book you can trust and rely on for both the Sanskrit and the English. I sought to make my translation literal but readable, and have included nothing which is not found in the text. My desire is that it increases your understanding of Yoga.

Chapter One

The Vital Principle

ईश्वर उवाच ।
एकं ज्ञानं नित्यमाद्यन्तशून्यं नान्यत्किंचिद्वृत्ति वस्तु सत्यम् ।
यद्भेदोऽस्मिन्निन्द्रियोपाधिना वै ज्ञानस्यायं भासते नान्यथैव ॥ १

The Lord said, "There is one eternal true knowledge,
without beginning or end. No other real entity exists.
The diversity which is found in this world appears
through the imposition of the senses on knowledge and
for no other reason.

अथ भक्तानुरक्तो हि वक्ति योगानुशासनम् ।
ईश्वरः सर्वभूतानामात्ममुक्तिप्रदायकम् ॥ २
त्यक्त्वा विवादशीलानां मतं दुर्ज्ञानहेतुकम् ।
आत्मज्ञानाय भूतानामनन्यगतिचेतसाम् ॥ ३

Affectionate toward his devotees, the Lord, having cast
aside opinions born of the ignorance of sophists, shall now
pronounce a Yoga teaching that bestows liberation on the
selves of all beings, so that beings whose minds are set on
no other destiny may have knowledge of their selves.

सत्यं केचित्प्रशंसन्ति तपः शौचं तथापरे ।
क्षमां केचित्प्रशंसन्ति तथैव शममार्जवम् ॥ ४

Some praise truth and others asceticism and purity. Some praise patience and others equanimity and honesty.

केचिद्दानं प्रशंसन्ति पितृकर्म तथापरे ।
केचित्कर्म प्रशंसन्ति केचिद्वैराग्यमुत्तमम् ॥ ५

Some praise charity and others ancestor worship. Some praise action and some absolute indifference.

केचिद्गृहस्थकर्माणि प्रशंसन्ति विचक्षणाः ।
अग्निहोत्रादिकं कर्म तथा केचित्परं विदुः ॥ ६

Some wise men praise the rites of the householder and some say that rites such as the fire sacrifice are the best.

मन्त्रयोगं प्रशंसन्ति केचित्तीर्थानुसेवनम् ।
एवं बहून्युपायानि प्रवदन्ति हि मुक्तये ॥ ७

Some praise Mantra Yoga and pilgrimage. In this way, many means to liberation are taught.

एवं व्यवसिता लोके कृत्याकृत्यविदो जनाः ।
व्यामोहमेव गच्छन्ति विमुक्ताः पापकर्मभिः ॥ ८

People in the world who are thus certain in their knowledge of what is and what is not to be done are freed from their sins, but only end up deluded.

एतन्मतावलम्बी यो लब्ध्वा दुरितपुण्यके ।
विभ्रमत्यवशः सोऽत्र जन्ममृत्युपरम्पराम् ॥ ९

The man who follows such a doctrine incurs sin and merit, and wanders out of control here in this world through a series of lives and deaths.

अन्यैर्मतिमतां श्रेष्ठैस्तत्त्वालोकनतत्परैः ।
आत्मनो बहवः प्रोक्ता नित्याः सर्वगतास्तथा ॥ १०

The best of the others among the wise, intent on discovering what is real, say that selves are many, eternal, and omnipresent.

यद्यत्प्रत्यक्षविषयं तदन्यन्नास्ति चक्षते ।
कुतः स्वर्गादयः सन्तीत्यन्ये निश्चितमानसाः ॥ ११

Some, asking where things such as heaven are to be found, are convinced that there is nothing apart from the object of direct perception.

ज्ञानप्रवाहमित्यन्ये शून्यं केचित्परं विदुः ।
द्वावेव तत्त्वे मन्यन्तेऽपरे प्रकृतिपुरुषौ ॥ १२

Others believe in a stream of consciousness. Some proclaim emptiness as the ultimate. Others think that there are two fundamental principles: matter and spirit.

अत्यन्तभिन्नमतयः परमार्थपरांमुखाः ।
एवमन्ये तु संचिन्त्य यथामति यथाश्रुतम् ॥ 13
निरीश्वरमिदं प्राहुः सेश्वरं च जगत्परे ।
वदन्ति विविधैर्भेदैः सुयुक्त्या स्थितिकातराः ॥ 14

Holding very different beliefs, some people thus shun the Ultimate Reality and, thinking in accordance with their beliefs and what they have heard, they say that there is no God in the universe. Others say that there is. Those uncertain of their position cleverly argue diverse opinions.

एते चान्ये च मुनिभिः संज्ञाभेदाः पृथग्विधाः ।
शास्त्रेषु कथिता ह्येते लोकव्यामोहकारकाः ॥ 15

These and various other different ideas have been taught by sages in the sacred texts and they confuse people.

एतद्विवादशीलानां मतं वक्तुं न शक्यते ।
भ्रमन्त्यस्मिं जनाः सर्वे मुक्तिमार्गबहिष्कृताः ॥ 16

One cannot explain these doctrines of people devoted to argument. Everyone loses their way in them and is driven from the path to liberation.

आलोक्य सर्वशास्त्राणि विचार्य च पुनः पुनः ।
इदमेकं सुनिष्पन्नं योगशास्त्रं परं मतम् ॥ 17

On examining all the sacred texts and contemplating
them repeatedly, this one consummate teaching of Yoga
is held to be supreme.

यस्मिन् ज्ञाते सर्वमिदं ज्ञातं भवति निश्चितम् ।
अस्मिन्परिश्रमः कार्यः किमन्यच्छास्त्रभाषितम् ॥ 18

When it is understood, everything is sure to be understood. One should work hard at it. There is no need to
bother with what is taught in other sacred texts.

योगशास्त्रमिदं गोप्यमस्माभिः परिभाषितम् ।
सुभक्ताय प्रदातव्यं त्रैलोक्ये च महात्मने ॥ 19

This Yoga teaching, taught by me, is to be guarded
and given to the man in the three worlds who is truly
devout and noble.

कर्मकाण्डं ज्ञानकाण्डमिति वेदो द्विधा मतः ।
भवति द्विविधो भेदो ज्ञानकाण्डस्य कर्मणः ॥ 20

The Vedas are considered to have two parts: the action
section and the knowledge section. There is a twofold
division of the knowledge section and of the action section.

द्विविधं कर्मकाण्डं स्यान्निषेधविधिपूर्वकम् ।
निषिद्धकर्मकरणे पापं भवति निश्चितम् ।
विधिना कर्मकरणे पुण्यं भवति निश्चितम् ॥ 21

The twofold action section consists of prohibitions and
commands. By doing what is prohibited, sin occurs. By
doing what is commanded, good deeds take place.

त्रिविधो विधिकूटः स्यान्नित्यनैमित्तकाम्यतः ।
नित्येऽकृते किल्बिषं स्यात्काम्ये नैमित्तके फलम् ॥ 22

Commands are of three kinds: obligatory, occasional,
and optional. When an obligatory command is not
obeyed, sin is incurred. The observance of occasional
and optional commands brings rewards.

द्विविधं तु फलं ज्ञेयं स्वर्गो नरक एव च ।
स्वर्गो नानाविधश्चैव नरकोऽपि तथा पुनः ॥ 23

Rewards should be known to be of two kinds: heaven and
hell. Heaven has many varieties and so too does hell.

पुण्यकर्मणि वै स्वर्गो नरकः पापकर्मणि ।
कर्मबन्धमयी सृष्टिर्नान्यथा भवति ध्रुवम् ॥ 24

Heaven results from good deeds, hell from sins.
Creation consists of the chain of karma and is certainly
not otherwise.

जन्तुभिश्रानुभूयन्ते स्वर्गे नाना सुखानि च ।
नानाविधानि दुःखानि नरके दुःसहानि वै ॥ 25

Beings experience many different pleasures in heaven and
many different unbearable sorrows in hell.

पापकर्मवशाद्दुःखं पुण्यकर्मवशात्सुखम् ।
तस्मात्सुखार्थी विविधं पुण्यं प्रकुरुते ध्रुवम् ॥ 26

Through the power of sin there is sorrow; through the
power of good deeds, pleasure. Therefore, one who desires
pleasure must perform various types of good deeds.

पापभोगावसाने तु पुनर्जन्म भवेत्खलु ।
पुण्यभोगावसाने तु नान्यथा भवति ध्रुवम् ॥ 27

When the rewards of sin are over, one is born again; when
the rewards of good deeds are over, the very same thing is
sure to happen.

स्वर्गेऽपि दुःखसंभोगः परस्त्रीदर्शनादिषु ।
ततो दुःखमिदं सर्वं भवेन्नास्त्यत्र संशयः ॥ 28

Even in heaven one experiences suffering, such as when
one sees other men's wives, so everything in life is
suffering. There is no doubt about this.

तत्कर्म कल्पकैः प्रोक्तं पुण्यं पापमिति द्विधा ।

पुण्यपापमयो बन्धो देहिनां कर्मतो भवेत् ॥ 29

Thus karma is said by the teachers to be of two sorts: good and bad. As a result of karma, embodied selves are bound by the chain of good and bad deeds.

इहामुत्रफलद्वेषी सफलं कर्म संत्यजेत् ।
नित्यनैमित्तिकं सङ्गं त्यक्त्वा योगे प्रवर्तते ॥ 30

Scornful of rewards in this world or the next, one should renounce action that brings rewards. One makes a start in Yoga after giving up attachment to obligatory and occasional actions.

कर्मकाण्डस्य माहात्म्यं ज्ञात्वा योगी त्यजेत्सुधीः ।
पुण्यपापद्वयं त्यक्त्वा ज्ञानकाण्डे प्रवर्तते ॥ 31

Having understood the importance of the Vedas' action section, the wise yogi should renounce it. After renouncing both good and bad deeds, he makes a start on the Vedas' section on knowledge.

आत्मा वाऽरे तु द्रष्टव्यः श्रोतव्य इति च श्रुतिः ।
सा सेव्या तु प्रयत्नेन मुक्तिदा हेतुदायिनी ॥ 32

The Vedic saying[1] that the self is to be seen and heard should be zealously observed: it grants liberation and knowledge of the Ultimate Reality.

---

[1]Found at Brihadaranyaka Upanishad 2.4.5.

दुरितेषु च पुण्येषु यो धीवृत्तिं प्रचोदयात् ।
सोऽहं प्रवर्ते मत्तो जगत्सर्वं चराचरम् ॥ 33
सर्वं च दृश्यते मत्तः सर्वं च मयि लीयते ।
न तद्भिन्नोऽहमस्म्यस्मिन्मद्भिन्नं न तु किंचन ॥ 34

That which impels the workings of the mind into bad
and good acts is me. The entire universe, animate and
inanimate, comes from me. Everything is seen through
me. Everything comes to rest in me. I am no different
from it and nothing in this world is different from me.

जलपूर्णेष्वसंख्येषु शरावेषु यथा रवेर् ।
एकस्य भात्यसंख्यत्वं तद्भेदोऽत्र दृश्यते ॥ 35

In the same way that a single sun reflects innumerable
times in innumerable bowls full of water, so diversity is
seen in the world.

उपाधिषु शरावेषु या संख्या वर्तते परम् ।
सा संख्या भवति यथा रवौ चात्मनि तत्तथा ॥ 36

But just as there are as many suns as there are bowls,
so there are as many selves as there are conditions for
their appearance.

यथैकः कल्पकः स्वप्ने नानाविधतयेष्यते ।
जागरेऽपि तथाप्येकस्तथैव बहुधा जगत् ॥ 37

Just as in a dream the dreamer appears in many different ways but is one on awakening, so the universe appears to have many forms.

सर्पबुद्धिर्यथा रज्जौ शुक्तौ वा रजतभ्रमः ।
तद्वज्जगदिदं सर्वं विवृतं परमात्मनि ॥ 38

In the same way that one thinks a rope is a snake or mistakes mother-of-pearl for silver, so this entire universe is made manifest on the supreme self.

रज्जुज्ञानाद्यथा सर्पो मिथ्याभूतो निवर्तते ।
आत्मज्ञानात्तथा याति मिथ्याभूतमिदं जगत् ॥ 39

Just as cognition of the rope makes the fallacious snake disappear, so cognition of the self makes this fallacious universe vanish.

रौप्यभ्रान्तिरियं याति शुक्तिज्ञानाद्यथा खलु ।
जगद्भ्रान्तिरियं याति चात्मज्ञानात्सदा तथा ॥ 40

In the same way that the mistaken perception of silver disappears on the cognition of mother-of-pearl, so the mistaken perception of the world always disappears on cognition of the self.

यथा रज्जूरगभ्रान्तिर्भवेद्रेकवशाज्ज्ञनात् ।
तथा चेयं जगद्भ्रान्तिरध्यासकल्पनाज्ज्ञनात् ।

आत्मज्ञानाद्यथा नास्ति रज्जुज्ञानाद्भुजंगमः ॥ 41

Just as by smearing one's eyes with frog fat one mistakes a rope for a snake, so by smearing one's eyes with erroneous inference and imagination one perceives the world mistakenly. This mistaken perception of the world ceases to exist from cognition of the self in the same way that the snake ceases to exist from cognition of the rope.

यथा दोषवशाच्छुक्रः पीतो भवति नान्यथा ।
अज्ञानदोषादात्मापि जगद्भवति दुस्त्यजम् ॥ 42

Just as through a bodily fault, and not otherwise, white appears as yellow, so too does the fault of ignorance create the impression, hard to abandon, that the self is the world.

दोषनाशे यथा शुक्लो गृह्यते रोगिणा स्वयम् ।
शुद्धज्ञानात्तथाज्ञाननाशादात्मा तथाकृतः ॥ 43

Just as upon the elimination of a disease a patient automatically perceives white as a result of correct knowledge, so when ignorance is eliminated the self is made real.

कालत्रयेऽपि न यथा रज्जुः सर्पो भवेदिति ।
तथात्मा न भवेद्विश्वं गुणातीतो निरञ्जनः ॥ 44

Just as in the past, present, or future a rope cannot become a snake, so the self, which is beyond qualities and without adornment, cannot become the universe.

आगमापायिनोऽनित्या नाश्यत्वादीश्वरादयः ।
आत्मबोधेन केनापि शास्त्रादेतद्विनिश्चितम् ॥ 45

The Lord and other gods, because they can be destroyed,
come and go and are not eternal. Using knowledge of
the self, a certain person has discerned this from the
sacred texts.

यथा वातवशात्सिन्धावुत्पन्नाः फेनबुद्बुदाः ।
तथात्मनि समुद्भूतः संसारः क्षणभंगुरः ॥ 46

Just as bubbles of foam arise in the ocean through the
influence of the wind, so the fleetingly ephemeral world
of samsara appears in the self.

अभेदो भासते नित्यं वस्तुभेदो न भासते ।
द्वित्वत्रित्वादिभेदोऽयं भ्रमत्वे पर्यवस्यति ॥ 47

Unity exists forever; there is no division of anything. This
division into two, three, or more is nothing but a mistake.

यद्भूतं यच्च भाव्यं वै मूर्तामूर्तं तथैव च ।
सर्वमेवं जगदिदं विवृतं परमात्मनि ॥ 48

Everything that has been or will be, whether manifest or
not, has thus been revealed to be the supreme self.

कल्पकैः कल्पिता विद्या मिथ्याजाता मृषात्मिका ।

एतन्मूलं जगदिदं कथं सत्यं भविष्यति ॥ 49

The teachers have declared knowledge arisen from false principles to be useless. This world is founded thus—how can it be real?

चैतन्यात्सर्वमुत्पन्नं जगदेतच्चराचरम् ।
तस्मात्सर्वं परित्यज्य चैतन्यं तु समाश्रयेत् ॥ 50

All this world, animate and inanimate, has arisen from consciousness, so one should abandon it completely and take refuge in consciousness.

घटस्याभ्यन्तरे बाह्ये यथाकाशं प्रवर्तते ।
तथात्माभ्यन्तरे बाह्ये ब्रह्माण्डस्य प्रवर्तते ॥ 51

Just as space exists inside and outside a pot, so the self exists inside and outside the universe.

असंलग्नं यथाकाशं मिथ्याभूतेषु वस्तुषु ।
असंलग्नस्तथात्मा तु कार्यवर्गेषु नान्यथा ॥ 52

Just as space is not in contact with unreal objects, so the self is not in any way in contact with the whole range of its activities.

ईश्वरादिजगत्सर्वमात्मव्याप्तं समन्ततः ।
एकोऽस्ति सच्चिदानन्दः पूर्णो द्वैतविवर्जितः ॥ 53

The gods and everything else in the entire universe are totally pervaded by the self. It is one, it is truth, consciousness, and bliss, and it is whole and free of duality.

यस्मात्प्रकाशको नास्ति स्वप्रकाशो भवेत्ततः ।
स्वप्रकाशो यतस्तस्मादात्मा ज्योतिःस्वरूपकः ॥ 54

Since there is no illuminator, it illuminates itself. Because it illuminates itself, it has the form of light.

अवच्छेदो यतो नास्ति देशकालस्वरूपतः ।
आत्मनः सर्वथा तस्मादात्मा पूर्णो भवेत्खलु ॥ 55

Because the self is in no way limited by place, time, or shape, it is truly whole.

यस्मान्न विद्यते नाशः पंचभूतैर्वृथात्मकैः ।
तस्मादात्मा भवेन्नित्यः स्वेनानाश्यो भवेत्खलु ॥ 56

Since it is not destroyed by the five unreal elements, the self is eternal. It cannot be destroyed by itself.

यस्मात्तदन्यो नास्तीह तस्मादेकोऽस्ति सर्वदा ।
यस्मात्तदन्यो मिथ्या स्यादात्मा सत्यो भवेत्खलु ॥ 57

Because there is nothing in the world other than it, it is forever one. Because that which is other than it is false, the self alone is true.

अविद्याभूतसंसारे दुःखनाशः सुखं यतः ।
ज्ञानादाद्यन्तशून्यं स्यात्तस्मादात्मा भवेत्सुखम् ॥ 58

In samsara, which arises from ignorance, suffering
is destroyed through true knowledge, resulting in a
happiness without beginning or end. Therefore the self
is happiness.

यस्मान्नाशितमज्ञानं ज्ञानेन विश्वकारणम् ।
तस्मादात्मा भवेज्ज्ञानं ज्ञानं तस्मात्सनातनम् ॥ 59

Because ignorance, the cause of the world, is destroyed
by knowledge, the self is knowledge and therefore
knowledge is eternal.

कालतो विविधं विश्वं यदा चैव भवेदिदम् ।
तदैकोऽस्ति स एवात्मा कल्पनापथवर्जितः ॥ 60

And while this world becomes diverse with time, the self
is one and unimaginable.

बाह्यानि सर्वभूतानि विनाशं यान्ति कालतः ।
यतो वाचो निवर्तन्ते आत्मा द्वैतविवर्जितः ॥ 61

With time all external objects are destroyed; the self is
ineffable, free from duality.

न खं वायुर्न चाग्निश्च न जलं पृथिवी न च ।

नैतत्कार्यं नेश्वरादि पूर्णैकात्मा भवेत्खलु ॥ 62

Not space, not air, not fire, not water, not earth, not this world, not the Lord and other gods, but only the self is truly whole.

आत्मानमात्मना योगी पश्यत्यात्मनि निश्चितम् ।
सर्वसंकल्पसंन्यासी त्यक्तमिथ्याभवग्रहः ॥ 63

The yogi who has renounced all desires and given up attachment to illusory existence is sure to see the self in the self by means of the self.

आत्मनात्मनि चात्मानं दृष्ट्वानन्तं सुखात्मकम् ।
विस्मृत्य विश्वं रमते समाधेस्तीव्रतस्तथा ॥ 64

After seeing the eternal blissful self in the self by means of the self and forgetting the world, he takes intense delight in samadhi.

मायैव विश्वजननी नाश्या तत्त्वधिया परा ।
यदा नाशं समायाति विश्वं नास्ति तदा खलु ॥ 65

It is Maya who is the mother of the universe. She can be completely destroyed by one who knows the truth. When she is destroyed, the universe no longer exists.

हेयं सर्वमिदं यत्तु मायाविलसितं यतः ।

स्वतो न प्रीतिविषयस्तनुवित्तसुखात्मकः ॥ 66

All this is the play of Maya and is to be rejected, so the body, riches, and pleasure are, by their own nature, not to be delighted in.

अरिर्मित्रमुदासीनं त्रिविधं स्यादिदं जगत् ।
व्यवहारेषु नियतं दृश्यते नान्यथा पुनः ॥ 67

This world can be of three kinds: inimical, friendly, or indifferent. It is consistently seen to be thus in one's everyday dealings, and is not otherwise.

प्रियाप्रियादिभेदस्तु वस्तुष्वनियतः स्फुटम् ।
आत्मोपाधिवशादेव भवेत्पुत्रेऽपि नान्यथा ॥ 68

Distinctions such as agreeable or disagreeable are clearly not inherent in objects. Even in a son it is only through one's own suppositions, and not otherwise, that they are to be found.

मायाविलसितं विश्वं ज्ञात्वैव श्रुतियुक्तिः ।
अध्यारोपापवादाभ्यां लयं कुर्वन्ति योगिनः ॥ 69

As soon as yogis realize from the arguments of the sacred texts that they have made incorrect assumptions about the universe and that it is the play of Maya, they use refutation to make it disappear.

कर्मजन्यमिदं विश्वं मत्वा कर्माणि वेदतः ।
निखिलोपाधिहीनो वै यदा भवति पुरुषः ।
तदा विजयतेऽखण्डज्ञानरूपी निरञ्जनः ॥ 70

This universe arises from action. When a man thinks
about his actions according to the Vedas and becomes
free of all supposition, he reigns supreme, takes the form
of complete knowledge, and is pure.

स हि कामयते सर्वं सृजते च प्रजाः स्वयम् ।
अविद्या भासते यस्मात्तस्मान्मिथ्या स्वभावतः ॥ 71

It is man who wills everything and he produces offspring
automatically. Ignorance appears from him, so he is
inherently false.

शुद्धब्रह्मणि संबन्धोऽविद्यया सह यो भवेत् ।
ब्रह्म तेनेशतां याति तत आभासते नभः ॥ 72

The conjunction of the pure Brahman with ignorance
results in Brahman becoming the Lord, and from him
space appears.

तस्मात्प्रकाशते वायुर्वायोरग्निस्ततो जलम् ।
प्रकाशते ततः पृथ्वी कल्पनेयं स्थिता सती ॥ 73

From that appears air; from air, fire; from that, water.
Earth appears from that. This is how creation works.

आकाशाद्वायुराकाशपवनादग्निसंभवः ।
खवाताग्रेर्जलं व्योमवाताग्निवारितो मही ॥ 74

From space arises air; from space and air, fire; from space,
air, and fire, water; from space, air, fire, and water, earth.

खं शब्दलक्षणं वायुश्चंचलः स्पर्शलक्षणः ।
स्याद्रूपलक्षणं तेजः सलिलं रसलक्षणम् ॥ 75
गन्धलक्षणिका पृथ्वी नान्यथा भवति ध्रुवम् ।
विशेषगुणाः स्फुरन्ति यतः शास्त्रादि्वनिर्णयः ॥ 76

Space is characterized by sound. Air moves and is characterized by touch. Fire is characterized by form. Water
is characterized by taste. Earth is characterized by smell.
They are definitely not otherwise. Particular attributes
are evident, as is ascertained from the sacred texts.

शब्दैकगुणमाकाशं द्विगुणो वायुरुच्यते ।
तथैव त्रिगुणं तेजो भवन्त्यापश्चतुर्गुणाः ॥ 77

Space has one attribute, that of sound. Air is said to have
two attributes, fire has three attributes, and water has
four attributes.

शब्दः स्पर्शश्च रूपं च रसो गन्धस्तथैव च ।
एतत्पंचगुणा पृथ्वी कल्पकैः कल्प्यतेऽधुना ॥ 78

Sound, touch, form, taste, and smell: earth is now
declared by the teachers to have these five attributes.

चक्षुषा गृह्यते रूपं गन्धो घ्राणेन गृह्यते ।
रसो रसनया स्पर्शस्त्वचा संगृह्यते परम् ।
श्रोत्रेण गृह्यते शब्दो नियतं भाति नान्यथा ॥ 79

Form is perceived by the eye, smell by the nose, taste by
the tongue, touch by the skin, and sound by the ear. This
is definitely how it is. It is not otherwise.

चैतन्यात्सर्वमुत्पन्नं जगदेतच्चराचरम् ।
अस्ति चेत्कल्पनेयं स्यान्नास्ति चेदस्ति चिन्मयम् ॥ 80

All this world, animate and inanimate, has arisen from
consciousness. To the extent that it exists, it is imagined;
as something nonexistent, it consists of consciousness.

पृथ्वी शीर्णा जले मग्ना जलं मग्नं च तेजसि ।
लीनं वायौ तथा तेजो व्योम्नि वातो लयं ययौ ।
अविद्यायां महाकाशो लीयते परमे पदे ॥ 81

Earth falls away and disappears in water. Water is
destroyed in fire. Fire vanishes in air. Air is absorbed into
space. The great space dissolves in ignorance, which disappears in the ultimate abode.

विक्षेपावरणाशक्तिर्दुरात्मा सुखरूपिणी ।
जडरूपा महामाया रजःसत्त्वतमोगुणा ॥ 82

Mahamaya has the powers of projection and concealment. She is evil natured and takes the form of happiness. She appears inert and has rajas, sattva, and tamas as attributes.

सा मायावरणाशक्त्यावृता विज्ञानरूपिणी ।
दर्शयेज्जगदाकारं तं विक्षेपस्वभावतः ॥ 83

Veiled by the power of concealment, that Maya has the form of intelligence. She makes the world appear through her innate power of projection.

तमोगुणाधिका विद्या या सा दुर्गा भवेत्स्वयम् ।
ईश्वरस्तदुपहितं चैतन्यं तद्भूद् ध्रुवम् ॥ 84

The wisdom goddess in which tamas is predominant is Durga herself. The consciousness connected with her is without doubt the Lord.

सत्वाधिका च या विद्या लक्ष्मी स्याद्दिव्यरूपिणी ।
चैतन्यं तदुपहितं विष्णुर्भवति नान्यथा ॥ 85

The wisdom goddess in which sattva is predominant is the beautiful Lakshmi. The consciousness connected with her is none other than Vishnu.

रजोगुणाधिका विद्या ज्ञेया सा वै सरस्वती ।
यश्चित्स्वरूपो भवति ब्रह्मा तदुपधारकः ॥ 86

The wisdom goddess in which rajas is predominant is Sarasvati. The consciousness connected with her is Brahma.

ईशाद्याः सकला देवा दृश्यन्ते परमात्मनि ।
शरीरादि जडं सर्वमविद्या कल्पिता तथा ॥ 87

The Lord and all the other gods together with the body and all other inanimate things are seen in the supreme self. Ignorance is designated thus.

एवंरूपेण कल्पन्ते कल्पका विश्वसंभवम् ।
तत्त्वातत्त्वा भवन्तीह कल्पनान्येन चोदिता ॥ 88

The teachers declare the origin of the universe to be like this. Someone else has proposed the hypothesis that both real and unreal objects exist in the world.

प्रमेयत्वादिरूपेण सर्वं वस्तु प्रकाश्यते ।
तथैव वस्तु नास्त्येव भासको वर्तते परम् ॥ 89

Every object is revealed through the appearance of qualities such as limitation. Thus the object does not exist. That which makes it appear does exist, however.

स्वरूपत्वेन रूपेण स्वरूपं वस्तु भासते ।
विशेषशब्दोपादाने भेदो भवति नान्यथा ॥ 90

Because it has its own form, an object appears in its own
form. There is differentiation only when a qualifying
word is applied.

एकः सत्यः पूरितानन्दरूपः पूर्णो व्यापी वर्तते नास्ति किंचित् ।
एतज्ज्ञानं यः करोत्येव नित्यं मुक्तः स स्यान्मृत्युसंसारदुःखात् ॥ ९१

There is nothing except that which is one, true, blissful,
whole, and all-pervading. He who realizes this is eternally
free from the sorrow of death and transmigration.

अध्यारोपापवादाभ्यां यत्र सर्वे लयं गताः ।
स एको वर्तते नान्यत्तच्चित्तेनावधार्यते ॥ ९२

That into which all things vanish, by means of realizing
that they have been incorrectly understood and dismissing them, is one and alone. It is grasped by the mind.

पितुरन्नमयात्कोशाज्जायते पूर्वकर्मतः ।
शरीरं वै विदुर्दुःखं स्वप्राग्भोगाय सुन्दरे ॥ ९३

The body is born of the material body of the father as a
result of past karma. It is for reaping the fruits of one's
past and is deemed unpleasant, O beautiful lady.

मांसास्थिस्नायुमज्जादिनिर्मितं भोगमन्दिरम् ।
केवलं दुःखभोगाय नाडीसन्ततिगुल्फितम् ॥ ९४

The locus of the reaping of rewards, it is a conglomeration of countless vessels, fashioned from flesh, bone, sinew, marrow, and other constituents, for the sole purpose of experiencing suffering.

परप्रेष्यमिदं गात्रं पंचभूतविनिर्मितम् ।
ब्रह्माण्डसंज्ञकं दुःखसुखभोगाय कल्पितम् ॥ 95

This body is the servant of another, composed of the five elements, known as the egg of Brahma and created to experience suffering and happiness.

बिन्दुः शिवो रजः शक्तिरुभयोर्मेलनात्स्वयम् ।
स्वप्नभूतानि जायन्ते स्वशक्त्या जडरूपया ॥ 96

Shiva is bindu, Shakti is rajas. From the union of the two, illusory elements arise spontaneously through the power of Maya.

तत्पंचीकरणात्स्थूलान्यसंख्यानि च कामतः ।
ब्रह्माण्डस्थानि वस्तूनि यत्र जीवोऽस्ति कर्मभिः ।
तद्भूतपंचकात्सर्वं भोगाय जीवसंज्ञिनाम् ॥ 97

And by making them into five, countless gross objects arise at will in the egg of Brahma, among which, according to its actions, is the jiva. Everything arises from those five elements so that those things called jiva may reap the fruits of their actions.

पूर्वकर्मानुरोधेन करोमि घटनामहम् ।
अजडः सर्वभूतान्वै जडस्थित्या भुनक्ति तान् ॥ 98

I make creation according to past actions. In a state of
nonsentience, the sentient experiences all the elements.

जडात्स्वकर्मभिर्बद्ध्वा जीवाख्यो विविधो भवेत् ।
भोगायोत्पद्यते सोऽपि ब्रह्माण्डाख्ये पुनः पुनः ।
जीवश्च लीयते भोगावसाने च स्वकर्मणः ॥ 99

Having taken shape out of insentient matter as a result
of its actions, that which goes by the name jiva assumes
various forms. It is born over and over again in that
which is called Brahma's egg in order to reap its rewards.
When it has finished reaping the rewards of its actions,
the jiva disappears."

इति श्रीशिवसंहितायां योगशास्त्रे ईश्वरपार्वतीसंवादे
प्रथमः पटलः ॥

Thus ends the first chapter in the glorious *Shiva Samhita*,
a treatise on Yoga in the form of a dialogue between the
Lord and Parvati.

द्वितीयः पटलः

Chapter Two

Knowledge

ईश्वर उवाच ।
देहेऽस्मिन्वर्तते मेरुः सप्तद्वीपसमन्वितः ।
सरितः सागरास्तत्र क्षेत्राणि क्षेत्रपालकाः ॥ 1

The Lord said, "In this body are Meru[1] and the seven
islands. On them are rivers, oceans, realms, and rulers.

ऋषयो मुनयः सर्वे नक्षत्राणि ग्रहास्तथा ।
पुण्यतीर्थानि पीठानि वर्तन्ते पीठदेवताः ॥ 2

There are seers, sages, all the constellations and planets,
sacred sites, shrines, and their attendant deities.

सृष्टिसंहारकर्तारौ भ्रमन्तौ शशिभास्करौ ।
नभो वायुश्च वह्निश्च जलं पृथ्वी तथैव च ॥ 3

The moon and sun, which bring about creation and
destruction, are revolving. There are space, air, fire, water,
and earth too.

---

[1]Mount Meru is the mythical mountain at the center of the universe. Its physical
homologue is the spine.

त्रैलोक्ये यानि भूतानि तानि सर्वाणि देहतः ।
मेरुं संवेष्ट्य सर्वत्र व्यवहारः प्रवर्तते ॥ ४

All the beings in the three worlds are found in the body.
Their usual activities take place everywhere around Meru.

जानाति यः सर्वमिदं स योगी नात्र संशयः ॥ ५

One who knows all this is certainly a yogi.

ब्रह्माण्डसंज्ञके देहे यथादेशं व्यवस्थितः ।
मेरुशृंगे सुधारश्मिर्द्विरष्टकलया युतः ।
वर्तते अहर्निशं सोऽपि सुधां वर्षत्यधोमुखः ॥ ६

In the body, which is called the egg of Brahma, the
nectar-rayed moon with its sixteen digits is in the appropriate place—on Meru's peak. It is there day and night,
facing downwards, raining nectar.

ततोऽमृतं द्विधाभूतं याति सूक्ष्मं यथा च वै ।
इडामार्गेण पुष्ट्यर्थं याति मन्दाकिनी जलम् ॥ ७

From there the subtle nectar of immortality becomes two
and flows forth. The Ganga water goes through Ida to
nourish the body.

पुष्णाति सकलं देहमिडामार्गेण निश्रितम् ।
एष पीयूषरश्मिर्हि वामपार्श्वे व्यवस्थितः ॥ ८

Going by way of Ida, it certainly does nourish the entire body. This ray of nectar is on the left side.

अपरः शुद्धदुग्धाभो हठात्कर्षति मण्डलात् ।
मध्यमार्गेण सृष्ट्यर्थं मेरौ संयाति चन्द्रमाः ॥ ९

The other looks like pure milk and draws forcefully on the orb. The moon enters Meru by way of the the central path in order to bring about creation.

मेरुमूले स्थितः सूर्यः कलाद्वादशसंयुतः ।
दक्षिणे पथि रश्मिभिर्वहत्यूर्ध्वं प्रजापतिः ॥ १०

The sun, with its twelve digits, is situated at the base of Meru. The lord of creatures, it uses its rays to journey upwards along the right-hand path.

पीयूषरश्मिनिर्यासं धातूंश्च ग्रसति ध्रुवम् ।
समीरमण्डले सूर्यो भ्रमते सर्वविग्रहे ॥ ११

It constantly consumes the nectar emitted by the moon and the constituents of the body. The sun wanders about the whole body in the sphere of the wind.

एषा सूर्यपरामूर्तिः निर्वाणं दक्षिणे पथि ।
वहते लग्नयोगेन सृष्टिसंहारकारकः ॥ १२

This other form of the sun carries nirvana along the right-hand path. By means of auspicious conjunctions, it brings about creation and destruction.

सार्धलक्षत्रयं नाड्यः सन्ति देहान्तरे नृणाम् ।
प्रधानभूता नाड्यस्तु तासु सन्ति चतुर्दश ॥ 13
सुषुम्णेडा पिंगला च गान्धारी हस्तिजिह्विका ।
कुहूः सरस्वती पूषा शंखिनी च पयस्विनी ॥ 14
वारुण्यलम्बुषा चैव विश्वोदरी यशस्विनी ।
एतासु तिस्रो मुख्याः स्युः पिंगलेडा सुषुम्णिका ॥ 15

There are three and one-half lakh nadis in the human body. Of these, fourteen are the most important: Sushumna, Ida, Pingala, Gandhari, Hastijihvika, Kuhu, Sarasvati, Pusha, Shankhini, Payasvini, Varuni, Alambusha, Vishvodari, and Yashasvini. Of these, three are preeminent: Pingala, Ida, and Sushumna.

तिसृष्वेका सुषुम्णैव मुख्या योगीन्द्रवल्लभा ।
अन्यास्तदाश्रयं कृत्वा नाड्यः सन्ति हि देहिनाम् ॥ 16

Of the three, Sushumna is the most important, the sweetheart of master yogis. The other nadis in embodied beings are connected to her.

नाड्यस्तु अधोवदनाः पद्मतन्तुनिभाः स्थिताः ।
पृष्ठवंशं समाश्रित्य सोमसूर्याग्निरूपिणी ॥ 17

The three nadis face downwards and resemble lotus fibers.
They are joined to the spinal column and take the form
of the moon, the sun, and fire.

तासां मध्यगता नाडी चित्रा स्यान्मम वलभा ।
ब्रह्मरन्ध्रं च तत्रैव सूक्ष्मात्सूक्ष्मतरं मतम् ॥ 18

In their middle is the Chitra nadi. She is beloved of me.
In her is the aperture of Brahman, which is considered to
be extremely subtle.

पंचवर्णोज्ज्वला शुद्धा सुषुम्णामध्यचारिणी ।
देहस्योपाधिरूपा सा सुषुम्णाभिन्नरूपिणी ॥ 19

Resplendent in five colors, she is pure, goes through the
middle of Sushumna, is the substrate of the body, and has
a different appearance from Sushumna.

दिव्यमार्गमिदं प्रोक्तममृतानन्दकारकम् ।
ध्यानमात्रेण योगीन्द्रो दुरितौघं विनाशयेत् ॥ 20

This divine path is said to bestow immortality and bliss.
Merely by meditating on it a master yogi destroys
all his sins.

गुदात्तु द्व्यंगुलादूर्ध्वं मेढ्राधो द्व्यंगुलात्परम् ।
चतुरंगुलविस्तारमाधारं वर्तते समम् ॥ 21

Two fingers above the anus, two fingers below the penis, four fingers broad, and flat, is the Adhara.

तस्मिन्नाधारपद्मे तु कर्णिकायां सुशोभना ।
त्रिकोणा वर्तते योनिः सर्वतन्त्रेषु गोपिता ॥ 22

In the pericarp of that Adhara lotus is a very beautiful triangular yoni,[2] kept secret in all the tantras.

तत्र विद्युल्लताकारा कुण्डली परदेवता ।
सार्द्धत्रिकरा कुटिला सूक्ष्मा भुजगसंनिभा ॥ 23

The great goddess Kundalini is there, in the form of a streak of lightning. Coiled three and one-half times, she is delicate and resembles a snake.

जगत्संसृष्टिरूपा सा निर्माणे सततोद्यता ।
वाचामवाच्या वाग्देवी सदा देवैर्नमस्कृता ॥ 24

She appears as the creation of the world and is always busy creating. Ineffable, she is the goddess of speech, constantly worshipped by the gods.

इडानाम्री तु या नाडी वाममार्गे व्यवस्थिता ।
मध्यनाडीं समाश्लिष्य वामनासापुटे गता ॥ 25

---

[2]Yoni literally means womb or vagina. In yogic subtle physiology it means a seat of the feminine creative energy.

The nadi called Ida is in the left path. Clinging to the central nadi, she goes to the left nostril.

पिंगला नाम या नाडी दक्षमार्गे व्यवस्थिता ।
सुषुम्णां सा समाश्लिष्य दक्षनासापुटे गता ॥ 26

The nadi called Pingala is in the right path. Clinging to Sushumna, she goes to the right nostril.

इडापिंगलयोर्मध्ये सुषुम्णा या भवेत्खलु ।
षड्सु स्थानेषु षट्चक्रं षट्पद्मं योगिनो विदुः ॥ 27

Between Ida and Pingala is Sushumna. Yogis teach there to be six chakras with six lotuses in the six stations.

पंचस्थानं सुषुम्णाया नामानि स्युर्बहूनि च ।
प्रयोजनवशात्तानि ज्ञातव्यानीह शास्त्रके ॥ 28

Sushumna has five stations and many names depending on her purpose. They are to be learnt from this text.

अन्या यास्त्यपरा नाडी मूलाधारात्समुत्थिता ।
रसनामेढ्रनयनं पादांगुष्ठं च श्रोत्रकम् ॥ 29
कुक्षिकक्षांगुष्ठवर्णं सर्वांङ्गं पायुकोशकम् ।
लब्ध्वा निवर्तते सा वै यथादेशसमुद्भवा ॥ 30

There is another lesser nadi arising from the Muladhara which reaches all over the body—to the tongue, the penis, the eyes, the big toes, the ears, the abdomen, the armpits, the thumbs, the anus, the scrotum—and returns to where it started.

एताभ्य एव नाडीभ्यः शाखोपशाखतः क्रमात् ।
सार्धलक्षत्रयं जातं यथाभागं व्यवस्थितम् ॥ 31

From these nadis and their branches and twigs, three and one-half lakh nadis arise in turn, fixed in their positions.

एता भोगवहा नाड्यो वायुसंचारदक्षकाः ।
ओताः प्रोताश्च संव्याप्य तिष्ठन्त्यस्मिन्कलेवरे ॥ 32

These nadis carry sensations and are capable of conducting the winds. They run across and along the body, pervading it.

सूर्यमण्डलमध्यस्थः कलाद्वादशसंयुतः ।
वस्तिदेशे ज्वलद्वह्निर्वर्तते चान्नपाचकः ॥ 33

In the region of the abdomen, at the middle of the orb of the sun and endowed with twelve digits, is a blazing fire which digests food.

वैश्वानरग्निरेषा वै मम तेजोंऽशसंभवः ।
करोति विविधं पाकं प्राणिनां देहमास्थितः ॥ 34

This Vaishvanara fire is born from a piece of my own fire. Situated in the bodies of living beings, it digests food in various ways.

आयुःप्रदायको वहिर्बलं पुष्टिं ददाति च ।
शरीरपाटवं चापि ध्वस्तरोगसमुद्भवः ॥ 35

Fire lengthens life, invigorates, and nourishes. It also quickens the body and brings about the destruction of disease.

तस्मादैश्वानराग्निं च प्रज्वाल्य विधिवत्सुधीः ।
तस्मिन्नन्नं हुनेद्योगी प्रत्यहं गुरुशिक्षया ॥ 36

Therefore the wise yogi should duly kindle the Vaishva-nara fire and sacrifice food into it every day according to the instructions of his guru.

ब्रह्माण्डसंज्ञके देहे स्थानानि स्युर्बहूनि च ।
मयोक्तानि प्रधानानि ज्ञातव्यानीह शास्त्रके ॥ 37

The body is known as Brahma's egg and in it are many stations. The important ones which need to be known have been taught by me here in this text.

नानाप्रकारनामानि स्थानानि विविधानि च ।
वर्तन्ते विग्रहे तानि कथितुं नैव शक्यते ॥ 38

The various stations in the body have many types and names. It is not possible to list them.

इत्थं प्रकल्पिते देहे जीवो वसति सर्वगः ।
अनादिवासनामालालंकृतः कर्मशृंखलः ॥ 39

In the body thus formed, the jiva resides everywhere. Adorned with a garland of beginningless desire, it is chained by karma.

नानाविधगुणोपेतः सर्वव्यापारकारकः ।
पूर्वार्जितानि कर्माणि भुनक्ति विविधानि च ॥ 40

It has many different attributes, performs all functions, and reaps the rewards of the various previously acquired karmas.

यद्यत्संदृश्यते लोके सर्वं तत्कर्मसंभवम् ।
सर्वकर्मानुसारेण जन्तुर्भोगान्भुनक्ति वै ॥ 41

Everything that is seen in the world results from karma. A living being reaps rewards according to all its karmas.

ये ये कामादयो दोषाः सुखदुःखप्रदायकाः ।
ते ते सर्वे प्रवर्तन्ते जीवे कर्मानुसारतः ॥ 42

Desire and all the other faults which bring about happiness and suffering arise in the jiva according to karma.

पुण्योपरक्तचैतन्यं प्राणान्प्रीणाति केवलम् ।
बाह्ये पुण्यमयं प्राप्य भोज्यवस्तु स्वयं भवेत् ॥ 43

Only a consciousness colored by merit makes for a happy
life. In the external world, things that are to be enjoyed
reach the meritorious and become theirs automatically.

ततः कर्मबलात्पुंसः सुखं वा दुःखमेव च ।
पापोपरक्तचैतन्यं नैव तिष्ठति निश्चितम् ॥ 44

So it is through the power of karma that a man is either
happy or suffers. A consciousness colored by sin is sure
not to remain.

न तद्भिन्नो भवेत्सोऽपि तद्भिन्नं न तु किंचन ।
मायोपहितचैतन्यात्सर्वं वस्तु प्रजायते ।
यथाकालोपभोगाय जन्तूनां विविधोद्भवः ॥ 45

And he is not separate from Brahman. Nothing is separate
from Brahman. All things arise from consciousness
conditioned by Maya. The various creatures arise to reap
their rewards at the appropriate time.

यथा दोषवशाच्छुक्तौ रजतारोपणं भवेत् ।
तथा स्वकर्मदोषाद्वै ब्रह्मण्यारोप्यते जगत् ॥ 46

Just as one can mistakenly consider mother-of-pearl to be
silver, so, through the fault of one's karma, Brahman can
be considered to be the universe.

सवासनाभ्रमोत्पन्नोन्मूलनातिसमर्थनम् ।
उत्पन्नं चेदीदृशं स्यज्ज्ञानं तन्मोक्षसाधनम् ॥ 47

Knowledge is more than capable of eradicating the
delusion that arises together with desires. Were such
knowledge to arise, it would be the means to liberation.

साक्षाद्विशेषदृष्टिस्तु साक्षात्कारिणि विभ्रमे ।
कारणं नान्यथा युक्त्या सत्यं सत्यं मयोदितम् ॥ 48

A particular way of seeing is clearly the cause of the mistaken perception of the agent of manifestation. It cannot
be argued to be otherwise. Truly, I have told you the truth.

साक्षात्कारिभ्रमे साक्षात्कारिणि नाशयेत्प्रमाः ।
सो हि नास्तीति संसारे भ्रमो नैव निवर्तते ॥ 49

When one is mistaken about the agent of manifestation,
with the result that the world is made manifest, one
destroys correct knowledge. When, in the world of
samsara, one has the idea that it is not that alone which
exists, then mistaken perception does not cease.

मिथ्याज्ञाननिवृत्तिस्तु विशेषदर्शनाङ्गवेत् ।
अन्यथा न निवृत्तिः स्याद्दृश्यते रजतभ्रमः ॥ 50

The cessation of wrong knowledge arises through special
sight. Otherwise it does not cease: there is the mistaken
perception of silver.

यावन्नोत्पद्यते ज्ञानं साक्षात्कारं निरञ्जनम् ।
तावत्सर्वाणि भूतानि दृश्यन्ते विविधानि वै ॥ 51

As long as clear-sighted and pure knowledge does not
arise, all objects are seen in their variety.

यदा कर्मार्जितं देहं निर्वाणसाधनं भवेत् ।
तदा शरीरवहनं सफलं स्यान्न चान्यथा ॥ 52

Only when the body acquired through karma is the
means to nirvana does having a body bear fruit.

यादृशी वासनामाला वर्तते जीवसंगिनी ।
तादृशं चरते जन्तुः कृत्याकृत्यविधौ भ्रमम् ॥ 53

The garland of desires that exists in connection with the
jiva is similar to the misunderstanding that a living being
has in its observance of what it should and should not do.

संसारसागरं तर्तुं यदीच्छेद्योगसाधकः ।
कृत्वा वर्णाश्रमं कर्म फलवर्जं तदाचरेत् ॥ 54

If an aspirant to Yoga wants to cross the ocean of samsara,
he should behave according to his caste and stage of life,
unattached to the fruits of his actions.

विषयासक्तपुरुषा विषयेषु सुखेप्सवः ।
वचोभिरुद्धनिर्वाणा वर्तन्ते पापकर्मणि ॥ 55

People who are attached to the objects of the senses and seek pleasure from them are prevented from reaching nirvana by words and abide in sin.

आत्मानमात्मना पश्यन्न किंचिदिह पश्यति ।
तदा कर्मपरित्यागे न दोषोऽस्ति मतं मम ॥ 56

Observing the self by means of the self, one sees nothing in this world. If one then gives up ritual action, there is, in my opinion, no transgression.

कामाद्यो विलीयन्ते ज्ञानादेव न चान्यथा ।
अभावे सर्वतत्त्वानां स्वयं तत्त्वं प्रकाशते ॥ 57

Vices such as desire disappear through knowledge and not otherwise. In the absence of all realities, Reality itself shines forth."

इति श्रीशिवसंहितायां योगशास्त्रे ईश्वरपार्वतीसंवादे
द्वितीयः पटलः ॥

Thus ends the second chapter in the glorious *Shiva Samhita*, a treatise on Yoga in the form of a dialogue between the Lord and Parvati.

Chapter Three

Practice

ईश्वर उवाच ।
हृद्यस्ति पंकजं दिव्यं दिव्यलिंगेन भूषितम् ।
कादिठान्ताक्षरोपेतं द्वादशारं विभूषितम् ॥ 1

The Lord said, "There is a divine lotus in the heart adorned with a heavenly linga.[1] It contains the syllables from *ka* to *ṭha*,[2] has twelve spokes and is beautiful.

प्राणो वसति तत्रैव वासनाभिरलंकृतः ।
अनादिकर्मसंश्लिष्टः प्रोक्तोऽहंकारसंयुतः ॥ 2

Prana resides right there. It is said to be adorned with desires, endowed with beginningless karma, and joined with the ego.

प्राणस्य वृत्तिभेदेन नामानि विविधानि च ।
वर्तन्ते तानि सर्वाणि कथितुं नैव शक्यते ॥ 3

---

[1]The linga is the penis and the symbol of Shiva.
[2]The syllables from *ka* to *ṭha* are *ka, kha, ga, gha, ṅa, ca, cha, ja, jha, ña, ṭa,* and *ṭha.*

Prana has various names according to its different activities. It is not possible to list them all.

प्राणोऽपानः समानश्चोदानो व्यानश्च पंचमः ।
नागः कूर्मश्च कृकरो देवदत्तो धनंजयः ॥ ४

Prana, apana, samana, udana, and vyana, the fifth; naga, kurma, krikara, devadatta, and dhananjaya.

दश नामानि मुख्यानि मयोक्तानीह शास्त्रके ।
कुर्वन्ते तेऽत्र कार्याणि प्रेरिताश्च स्वकर्मभिः ॥ ५

I have stated the ten main names here in this text. The winds perform their tasks in the body driven by their own karmas.

अत्रापि वायवः पंच मुख्याः स्युर्दशतः पुनः ।
तत्रापि श्रेष्ठकर्तारौ प्राणापानौ मयोदितौ ॥ ६

Furthermore, of those ten, five are chief, and of them, prana and apana are said by me to be the most important agents.

हृदि प्राणो गुदेऽपानः समानो नाभिमण्डले ।
उदानः कण्ठदेशे स्याद्व्यानः सर्वशरीरगः ॥ ७

Prana is in the heart, apana in the anus, samana in the region of the navel, udana in the region of the throat, and vyana pervades the body.

नागादिवायवः पंच कुर्वन्ति ते च विग्रहे ।
उद्गारोन्मीलनं क्षुत्तृड्जृम्भां हिक्कां च पंचमीम् ॥ ८

The five winds beginning with naga bring about the
following in the body: belching, opening the eyes, hunger
and thirst, yawning, and hiccuping, the fifth.

अनेन विधिना यो वै ब्रह्माण्डं वेत्ति विग्रहम् ।
सर्वपापविनिर्मुक्तः स वै याति परां गतिम् ॥ ९

He who thus knows the body to be the egg of Brahma is
freed from all sins and goes to the ultimate destination.

अधुना कथयिष्यामि क्षिप्रं योगस्य सिद्धये ।
यज्ज्ञात्वा नावासीदन्ति योगिनो योगसाधने ॥ १०

Now I shall quickly teach how to succeed in Yoga.
Yogis who know this do not fail in their practice of Yoga.

भवेद्वीर्यवती विद्या गुरुवक्त्रसमुद्भवा ।
अन्यथा फलहीना स्यान्निर्वीर्याप्यतिदुःखदा ॥ ११

If it comes from a guru's mouth, wisdom is potent. If
it does not, it is barren, it is impotent, and it brings
great suffering.

गुरुं सन्तोष्य यत्नेन यो वै विद्यामुपासते ।
अविलम्बेन विद्यायास्तस्याः फलमवाप्नुयात् ॥ १२

He who zealously makes his guru happy and is devoted to his wisdom quickly gains the reward of that wisdom.

गुरुः पिता गुरुर्माता गुरुर्देवो न संशयः ।
कर्मणा मनसा वाचा तस्माच्छिष्यैः प्रसेव्यते ॥ 13

The guru is the father, the guru is the mother, the guru is God. This is certain. As a result he is served by his pupils in thought, word, and deed.

गुरुप्रसादतः सर्वं लभ्यते शुभमात्मनः ।
तस्मात्सेव्यो गुरुर्नित्यमन्यथा न शुभं भवेत् ॥ 14

Everything that is good for the self is obtained through the grace of the guru, so the guru is to be served constantly, or else no good will happen.

प्रदक्षिणत्रयं कृत्वा स्पृष्ट्वा सव्येन पाणिना ।
अष्टांगेन नमस्कुर्यादनुरुपादसरोरुहम् ॥ 15

After walking clockwise around him three times, the yogi should touch his lotus feet with his right hand and prostrate himself before them.

श्रद्धयात्मवतां पुंसां सिद्धिर्भवति निश्चिता ।
अन्येषां च न सिद्धिः स्यात्तस्माद्यत्नेन साधयेत् ॥ 16

With faith, perfection is assured for those who are self-possessed. For others there will be no success, so one should practice zealously.

न भवेत्संगयुक्तानां तथाविश्वासिनामपि ।
गुरुपूजाविहीनानां तथा च बहुसंगिनाम् ॥ 17
मिथ्यावादरतानां च तथा निष्ठुरभाषिणाम् ।
गुरुसंतोषहीनानां न सिद्धिः स्यात्कदाचन ॥ 18

Perfection will never happen for those who are devoted to worldly attachments, who do not have faith, who do not worship their gurus, who are very social, who delight in lying, who speak harshly, and who do not please their gurus.

फलिष्यतीति विश्वासः सिद्धेः प्रथमलक्षणम् ।
द्वितीयं श्रद्धया युक्तं तृतीयं गुरुपूजनम् ॥ 19

The first mark of perfection is the conviction that one's practice will bear fruit. The second is having faith, the third is honoring one's guru.

चतुर्थं समताभावः पंचमेन्द्रियनिग्रहः ।
षष्ठं च प्रमिताहारः सप्तमं नैव विद्यते ॥ 20

The fourth is equanimity, the fifth restraint of the sense organs, and the sixth curbing of the diet. There is no seventh.

योगोपदेशं संप्राप्य लब्ध्वा योगविदं गुरुम् ।
गुरूपदिष्टविधिना धिया निश्चित्य साधयेत् ॥ 21

After finding a guru knowledgeable in Yoga and receiving instruction in Yoga, the yogi should carefully and resolutely practice in the way taught by the guru.

सुशोभने मठे योगी पद्मासनसमन्वितः ।
आसनोपरि संविश्य पवनाभ्यासमाचरेत् ॥ 22

In a beautiful hermitage the yogi should sit on a seat in Padmasana and practice breath exercises.

समकायः प्राञ्जलिश्च प्रणम्य च गुरुं सुधीः ।
दक्षे वामे च विघ्नेशं क्षेत्रपालाम्बिकां पुनः ॥ 23

His body straight and his palms together, the wise yogi should pay homage to his guru and then to Ganesha on the right side and Kshetrapala and Ambika on the left.

ततः स्वदक्षांगुष्ठेन निरुध्य पिंगलां सुधीः ।
इडया पूरयेद्वायुं यथाशक्त्या तु कुम्भयेत् ॥ 24

Then the wise yogi should block Pingala with his right thumb, inhale through Ida, and hold his breath for as long as he can.

ततस्त्यक्त्वा पिंगलया शनैरेव न वेगतः ।

पुनः पिंगलयापूर्य यथाशक्त्या च कुम्भयेत् ॥ 25

Then he should exhale through Pingala—gently, not
quickly—before inhaling through Pingala and holding
his breath for as long as he can.

इडया रेचयेद्धीमान्न वेगेन शनैः शनैः ।
एवं योगविधानेन कुर्याद्द्विंशति कुम्भकान् ॥ 26

He should exhale through Ida—gently, not quickly. Using
this method of Yoga he should do twenty kumbhakas.[3]

सर्वद्वन्द्वविनिर्मुक्तः प्रत्यहं विगतालसः ।
प्रातःकाले च मध्याह्ने च सूर्यास्ते चार्धरात्रके ।
कुर्यादेवं चतुर्वारं कालेष्वेतेषु कुम्भकान् ॥ 27

Energized and free from all dualities, he should practice
kumbhakas in this way four times every day at the
following junctures: dawn, midday, sunset, and midnight.

इत्थं मासत्रयं कुर्यादिनालस्यो दिने दिने ।
ततो नाडीविशुद्धिः स्यादविलम्बेन निश्चितम् ॥ 28

If he energetically practices thus every day for three
months, then his nadis are sure to be purified forthwith.

यदा तु नाडीशुद्धिः स्याद्योगिनस्तत्त्वदर्शिनः ।

---

[3]Kumbhaka is the holding of the breath.

तदा विध्वस्तपापस्य भवेदारंभसंभवः ॥ 29

When the nadis of the yogi who has beheld the Ultimate
Reality are purified, his sins are destroyed and the
arambha state arises in him.

चिह्नानि योगिनो देहे दृश्यन्ते नाडिशुद्धितः ।
कथ्यन्ते तु समन्तात्तान्यंगे संक्षेपतो मया ।
समकायः सुगन्धिश्च सुकान्तिः सुररसाधरः ॥ 30

Signs are seen in the yogi's body as a result of the purifi-
cation of the nadis. For your benefit, I shall list all these
physical signs in brief: he sits up straight, he is fragrant,
he is beautiful, and he is a receptacle for the nectar
of the gods.

आरम्भश्च घटश्चैव तथा परिचयस्तथा ।
निष्पत्तिः सर्वयोगेषु योगावस्था भवन्ति ताः ॥ 31

Arambha, ghata, parichaya, and then nishpatti: these
stages of Yoga arise in all Yogas.

आरम्भः कथितोऽस्माभिरधुना वायुसिद्धये ।
अपरः कथ्यते पश्चात्सर्वदुःखौघनाशकः ॥ 32

I have described arambha. Now, for the mastery of breath,
I shall describe the next, which results in the destruction
of all suffering and sin.

प्रौढवह्निः सुभोजी च सुखी सर्वाङ्गसुन्दरः ।
संपूर्णहृदयो योगी सर्वोत्साहबलान्वितः ।
जायन्ते योगिनोऽवश्यमेते सर्वे कलेवरे ॥ 33

The yogi has a strong digestive fire, eats well, is happy, has a beautiful body, is big hearted, and has great willpower and strength. All these signs are sure to arise in the body of the yogi.

अथ वर्ज्यं प्रवक्ष्यामि योगविघ्नकरं परम् ।
येन संसारदुःखाब्धिं तीर्त्वा यास्यन्ति योगिनः ॥ 34

Now I shall teach what is to be avoided, the great hindrances to Yoga, so that yogis can cross the ocean of the sorrows of samsara.

अम्लं रूक्षं तथा तीक्ष्णं लवणं सार्षपं कटु ।
बहु च भ्रमणं प्रातःस्नानं तैलं विदाहकम् ॥ 35
स्तेयं हिंसा परद्वेषं चाहंकारमनार्जवम् ।
उपवासमसत्यं च मोहं च प्राणिपीडनम् ॥ 36
स्त्रीसंगमग्निसेवां च बह्वालापं प्रियाप्रियम् ।
अतीवभोजनं योगी त्यजेदेतानि निश्चितम् ॥ 37

Sour, astringent, pungent, salty, mustard, and bitter flavors; too much walking, bathing in the early morning, burning oil, stealing, violence, hatred of others, pride, insincerity, fasting, untruthfulness, folly, cruelty to animals, the company of women, the use of fire, too much

chatter—whether good natured or not—and overeating:
the yogi should definitely give up these.

उपायं च प्रवक्ष्यामि क्षिप्रं योगस्य सिद्धये ।
गोपनीयं सुसिद्धानां येन सिद्धिर्भवेद् ध्रुवम् ॥ 38

I shall teach the means to quick success in Yoga, the
secret of the finest, perfected masters, by which perfection is sure to arise.

क्षीरं घृतं च मिष्टान्नं ताम्बूलं चूर्णवर्जितम् ।
कर्पूरं निस्तुषं पिष्टं सुमठं सूक्ष्मवस्त्रकम् ॥ 39
सिद्धान्तश्रवणं नित्यं वैराग्यं गृहसेवनम् ।
नामसंकीर्तनं विष्णोः सुनादश्रवणं परम् ॥ 40
धृतिः क्षमा तपः शौचं ह्रीर्मतिर्गुरुसेवनम् ।
सदैतानि परं योगी नियमानि समाचरेत् ॥ 41

Milk, ghee, sweets, betel without lime, camphor,
unhusked and ground food, a beautiful hermitage, fine
cloth, listening to philosophical discourses, constant
dispassion, domestic duties, singing the name of Vishnu,
listening to harmonious music, resolve, patience, austerity,
purity, modesty, understanding, and attendance upon
one's guru: the yogi should always practice these observances to the utmost.

अनिलेऽर्कप्रवेशे च भोक्तव्यं योगिभिः सदा ।
वायौ प्रविष्टे शशिनि शयनं साधकोत्तमैः ।

सद्यो भुक्तेऽपि क्षुधिते नाभ्यासः क्रियते बुधैः ॥ 42

Yogis should always eat when the wind has entered the sun. The best practitioners rest when the wind has entered the moon. The wise do not practice straight after eating or when hungry.

अभ्यासकाले प्रथमं कुर्यात्क्षीराज्यभोजनम् ।
ततोऽभ्यासे स्थिरीभूते न तादृङ्नियमग्रहः ॥ 43

At the time of practice, one should first eat milk and ghee. Then once the practice is established, this rule need not be observed.

अभ्यासिना च भोक्तव्यं स्तोकं स्तोकमनेकधा ।
पूर्वोक्तकालेषु कुर्यात्कुम्भकान्प्रतिवासरम् ॥ 44

The practitioner should eat small amounts frequently. He should practice kumbhakas daily at the aforementioned times.

ततो यथेष्टशक्तिः स्याद्योगिनो वायुधारणे ।
यथेष्टधारणाद्वायोः कुम्भकः सिध्यति ध्रुवम् ।
केवले कुम्भके सिद्धे किं न स्यादिह योगिनः ॥ 45

Then the yogi will be able to hold his breath for as long as he wants. Through being able to hold the breath for as long as he wants, kumbhaka is sure to be perfected.

When Kevalakumbhaka is perfected, nothing in the world is impossible for the yogi.

स्वेदः संजायते देहे योगिनः प्रथमोद्यमे ।
यदा संजायते स्वेदो मर्दनं कारयेत्सुधीः ।
अन्यथा विग्रहे धातुर्नष्टो भवति योगिनः ॥ 46

At the yogi's first attempts, sweat is produced on his body. When sweat is produced, the wise yogi should rub it in or the essential constituents of his body will be lost.

द्वितीये हि भवेत्कम्पो दार्दुरी मध्यमे मता ।
ततोऽधिकतराभ्यासाद्गगने साधकोऽधिकः ॥ 47

In the second stage there is trembling, in the middle stage the practitioner is said to jump about like a frog, and from further practice a good practitioner can fly.

योगी पद्मासनस्थोऽपि भुवमुत्सृज्य वर्तते ।
वायुसिद्धिस्तदा ज्ञेया संसारध्वान्तनाशिनी ॥ 48

When the yogi sitting in Padmasana leaves the ground, know that to be mastery of air, the destroyer of the darkness of samsara.

तावत्कालं प्रकुर्वीत योगोक्तनियमग्रहम् ।
अल्पनिद्रापुरीषं च स्तोकं मूत्रं च जायते ।
अरोगित्वमदीनत्वं योगिनस्तत्त्वदर्शिनः ॥ 49

One should observe the rules for Yoga that have been mentioned until sleep, defecation, and urination diminish. The yogi who experiences the ultimate reality is not ill or depressed.

स्वेदो लाला कृमिश्चैव सर्वथैव न जायते ।
कफपित्तानिलाश्चैव साधकस्य कलेवरे ॥ 50

Neither sweat, saliva, nor worms, nor imbalances of kapha, pitta, and vata arise in the body of the practitioner.

तस्मिन्काले साधकस्य भोज्येष्वनियमग्रहः ।
अत्यल्पं बहुधा भुक्त्वा योगी न व्यथते हि सः ॥ 51

Then the practitioner need not observe dietary restrictions. The yogi is not troubled if he eats very little or very much.

अभ्यासवशाद्योगी भूचरीसिद्धिमाप्नुयात् ।
येन दुर्धर्षजन्तूनां गतिः स्यात्पाणिताडनात् ॥ 52

Through the power of practice, the yogi obtains Bhuchari siddhi,[4] whereby he can move like the animals which are hard to catch when hands are clapped.

सन्त्यत्र बहवो विघ्नाः दारुणा दुर्निवारणाः ।
तथापि साधयेद्योगी प्राणैः कण्ठगतैरपि ॥ 53

---

[4]A siddhi is a magical power achieved through the perfection of a yoga practice.

In Yoga, there are a lot of fearsome obstacles that are hard to avoid, despite which the yogi should keep on striving, even if he is at his last gasp.

ततो रहस्युपाविष्टः साधकः संयतेन्द्रियः ।
प्रणवं प्रजपेद्दीर्घं विघ्नानां नाशहेतवे ॥ 54

Thereupon the practitioner, sitting in private with his sense organs restrained, should intone the syllable *om* in order to get rid of obstacles.

पूर्वार्जितानि कर्माणि प्राणायामेन निश्चितम् ।
नाशयेत्साधको धीमानिह लोकोद्भवानि च ॥ 55

By means of pranayama, the wise practitioner is sure to destroy all the karmas he has previously acquired and those which have arisen in this life.

पूर्वार्जितानि पापानि पुण्यानि विविधानि च ।
नाशयेत् षोडशप्राणायामेन योगिपुंगवः ॥ 56

The best yogi gets rid of the various good and bad deeds he has amassed in the past by means of sixteen pranayamas.

पापातुलाचलानाहो प्रदहेत्प्रलयाग्निना ।
ततः पापविनिर्मुक्तो योगी पुण्यानि नाशयेत् ॥ 57

Oh! He should burn his enormous mountains of sin with the doomsday fire. Then, free from sin, the yogi should destroy his store of merit.

प्राणायामेन योगीन्द्रो लब्ध्वैश्वर्याष्टकानि वै ।
पापपुण्योदधिं तीर्त्वा त्रैलोक्येश्वरतामियात् ॥ 58

By means of pranayama the lord amongst yogis attains the eight powers, crosses the ocean of sin and merit, and becomes the lord of the three worlds.

ततोऽभ्यासक्रमेणैव घटिकात्रितयं भवेत् ।
येन स्यात्सकला सिद्धिर्योगिनः स्वेप्सिता ध्रुवम् ॥ 59

Only by gradual practice can the yogi hold his breath for three ghatikas,[5] by which he is sure to get the complete success that he desires.

वाक्सिद्धिः कामचारित्वं दूरदृष्टिस्तथैव च ।
दूरश्रुतिः सूक्ष्मदृष्टिः परकायप्रवेशनम् ॥ 60
विण्मूत्रलेपेन स्वर्णमदृश्यकरणं तथा ।
भवन्त्येतानि महतां खेचरत्वं च योगिनाम् ॥ 61

Mastery of speech, the ability to go where he wants, long-distance vision and hearing, subtle sight, the ability to enter another's body, the power of producing gold

---

[5]One ghatika is twenty-four minutes.

by smearing objects with one's feces and urine, and the capacity to make things invisible—these, and the ability to move through space, arise in great yogis.

यदा भवेद्घटावस्था पवनाभ्यासिनः परा ।
तदा संसारचक्रेऽस्मिन्तन्नास्ति यन्न साधयेत् ॥ 62

When the great ghata stage arises for the practitioner of pranayama, then there is nothing that he cannot accomplish on the wheel of samsara.

प्राणापानौ नादबिन्दू जीवात्मपरमात्मनौ ।
मिलित्वा घटते यस्मात्तस्मादै घट उच्यते ॥ 63

It is called ghata because prana and apana, nada and bindu, and jivatma and paramatma come together and unite.[6]

याममात्रं यदा धर्तुं समर्थः स्यादतन्द्रितः ।
प्रत्याहारस्तदैव स्यान्नान्यथा भवति ध्रुवम् ॥ 64

Only when the yogi is able to hold the breath for one yama[7] without tiring does pratyahara arise. It definitely does not happen otherwise.

यद्यज्ज्ञानाति योगीन्द्रस्तत्तदस्मीति भावयेत् ।
यैरिन्द्रियैर्विधानज्ञस्तदिन्द्रियजयो भवेत् ॥ 65

---

[6]"Unite" is a translation of *ghaṭate*, hence the name ghata.
[7]A yama is three hours.

The lord of yogis should think 'I am that' of whatever he perceives. He gains mastery over whichever sense organ is used to understand this principle.

याममात्रं यदा पूर्णं भवेदभ्यासयोगतः ।
एकवारं प्रकूर्वीत तदा योगी च कुम्भकम् ॥ 66

When through application of the practice he can hold his breath for a full yama, then the yogi should practice kumbhaka once a day.

दण्डाष्टकं यदा वायुर्निश्चलो योगिनो भवेत् ।
स्वसामर्थ्यात्तदांगुष्ठे तिष्ठेद्वातूलवत्सुधीः ॥ 67

When the yogi's breath does not move for eight dandas,[8] then that wise man has the power to stand on his thumb as if he were made of air.

ततः परिचयावस्था योगिनोऽभ्यासतो भवेत् ।
यदा वायुश्चन्द्रसूर्यं त्यक्त्वा तिष्ठति निश्चलः ॥ 68

After this, with practice the yogi attains the stage of parichaya, when the breath leaves the sun and the moon and stays still.

---

[8]The length of a danda is unclear, but the sense suggests that eight dandas equal one yama. *Vātūla*, which has been translated as "made of air," can also mean "crazy" in the sense of one whose winds are deranged.

वायौ परिचितो वायुः सुषुम्णाव्योम्नि संचरेत् ।
क्रियाशक्तिं गृहीत्वैवं चक्रान्भित्वा च निश्चितम् ॥ 69

The breath heaped on breath[9] is sure to take hold of the
action shakti, pierce the chakras, and enter the space in
the Sushumna.

यदा परिचयावस्था भवेदभ्यासयोगतः ।
त्रिकूटं कर्मणां योगी तदा पश्यति निश्चितम् ॥ 70

When through application of the practice the parichaya
stage arises, the yogi is sure to see the three groups
of karma.

ततश्च कर्मकूटानि प्रणवेन विनाशयेत् ।
स योगी कर्मभोगाय कायव्यूहं समाचरेत् ॥ 71

He should then use the syllable *om* to destroy the groups
of karma. The yogi should prepare his body in such a way
that he can experience the results of his karma.

अस्मिन्काले महायोगी पंचधा धारणां चरेत् ।
येन भूरादिसिद्धिः स्यात्तत्तद्भूतभयापहा ॥ 72

Then the great yogi should practice the fivefold dharana,
by means of which he masters earth and the other
elements and has nothing to fear from any of them.

---

[9]Parichaya means "heaping up," "accumulation."

आधारे घटिकाः पंच लिंगस्थाने तथैव च ।
तदूर्ध्व घटिकाः पंच नाभिहृन्मध्यके तथा ॥ 73
भूमध्योर्ध्वं तथा पंचघटिका धारयेत्सुधीः ।
तथा भूरादिना नष्टो योगीन्द्रो न भवेत्खलु ॥ 74

The wise yogi should practice dharana for five ghatikas on
the Adhara, the same on the place of the penis, for five
ghatikas on the region above there, and likewise on the
area between the navel and the heart, and for five ghatikas
above the center of the eyebrows. The lord of yogis
cannot then be destroyed by earth and the other elements.

मेधावी पंचभूतानां धारणां यः समभ्यसेत् ।
शतब्रह्ममृतेनापि मृत्युस्तस्य न विद्यते ॥ 75

The wise yogi who practices dharana of the five elements
does not die even in a hundred deaths of Brahma.

ततोऽभ्यासक्रमेणैव निष्पत्तिर्योगिनो भवेत् ।
अनादिकर्मबीजानि येन तीर्त्वामृतं पिबेत् ॥ 76

Only by gradual practice does the yogi reach the nishpatti
stage, by which he escapes the seeds of beginningless
karma and drinks the nectar of immortality.

यदा निष्पत्तिसंपन्नः समाधिः स्वेच्छया भवेत् ॥ 77
गृहीत्वा चेतनां वायुः क्रियाशक्तिं च वेगवान् ।
सर्वाश्चक्रान्विजित्वाशु ज्ञानशक्तौ विलीयते ॥ 78

When samadhi automatically arises together with nishpatti, the impetuous breath takes hold of conscious-ness and the action shakti, hurries through all the chakras, and comes to rest in the knowledge shakti.

इदानीं क्लेशहान्यर्थं वक्तव्यं वायुसाधनम् ।
येन संसारचक्रेऽस्मिन्नरोगहानिर्भवेद् ध्रुवम् ॥ 79

In order to remove problems, the technique of mastering the breath is now to be taught, by which diseases are sure to be destroyed on this wheel of samsara.

रसनां तालुमूले यः स्थापयित्वा विपश्चितः ।
पिबेत्प्राणानिलं तस्य रोगाणां संक्षयो भवेत् ॥ 80

For the wise yogi who fixes his tongue at the root of the palate and drinks prana, there is complete elimination of his diseases.

काकचंच्वा पिबेद्वायुं शीतलं यो विचक्षणः ।
प्राणापानविधानज्ञः स भवेन्मुक्तिभाजनः ॥ 81

The clever yogi, who drinks in cool air with his mouth in the shape of a crow's beak and knows the operations of prana and apana, becomes a worthy recipient of liberation.

सरसं यः पिबेद्वायुं प्रत्यहं विधिना सुधीः ।
नश्यन्ति योगिनस्तस्य श्रमदाहज्वरामयाः ॥ 82

For the wise yogi who duly drinks air and nectar every day, fatigue, fever, old age, and illness are no more.

रसनामूर्ध्वगां कृत्वा यश्चन्द्रसलिलं पिबेत् ।
मासमात्रेण योगीन्द्रो मृत्युं जयति निश्चितम् ॥ 83

The lord among yogis, who turns his tongue upwards and drinks the liquid from the moon, is sure to conquer death within just one month.

राजदन्तबिलं गाढं संपीड्य विधिना पिबेत् ।
ध्यात्वा कुण्डलिनीं देवीं षण्मासेन कविर्भवेत् ॥ 84

He should tightly press the aperture at the uvula and drink correctly. Meditating on the goddess Kundalini, he becomes a sage within six months.

काकचंच्वा पिबेद्वायुं सन्ध्ययोरुभयोरपि ।
कुण्डलिन्याः मुखे ध्यात्वा क्षयरोगस्य शान्तये ॥ 85

To alleviate a wasting disease, he should drink in air at the beginning and end of the day with his mouth in the shape of a crow's beak, visualizing the air at Kundalini's mouth.

अहर्निशं पिबेद्योगी काकचंच्वा विचक्षणः ।
दूरश्रुतिर्दूरदृष्टिस्तथा स्यादर्शनं खलु ॥ 86

With his mouth shaped like a crow's beak, the wise
yogi should breathe in air day and night. Long distance
hearing and sight arise, together with discernment.

दन्तैर्दन्तान्समापीड्य पिबेद्वायुं शनैः शनैः ।
ऊर्ध्वजिह्वः सुमेधावी मृत्युं जयति सोऽचिरात् ॥ 87

Pressing his teeth together, he should drink in air very
gently. With his tongue turned upwards, the wise yogi
quickly conquers death.

षण्मासमात्रमभ्यासं यः करोति दिने दिने ।
सर्वपापविनिर्मुक्तो रोगान्नाशयते हि स ॥ 88

He who practices it every day for just six months is freed
from all sin and gets rid of diseases.

संवत्सरकृताभ्यासान्मृत्युं जयति निश्चितम् ।
तस्मादतिप्रयत्नेन साधयेत्साधकोत्तमः ॥ 89

By practicing for a year he is sure to conquer death. Therefore the best of practitioners should practice zealously.

वर्षत्रयकृताभ्यासाद्भैरवो भवति ध्रुवम् ।
अणिमादिगुणान् लब्ध्वा जितभूतगणः स्वयम् ॥ 90

After three years of practice he is sure to become Bhairava.
He obtains the powers of becoming infinitesimal and so
forth and automatically conquers all the elements.

रसनामूर्ध्वगां कृत्वा क्षणार्धं यदि तिष्ठति ।
क्षणेन मुच्यते योगी व्याधिमृत्युजरादिभिः ॥ 91

If he turns his tongue upwards and remains thus for half
an instant, the yogi is quickly freed from diseases, death,
and decrepitude.

रसनां प्राणसंयुक्तां पीड्यमानां विचिन्तयेत् ।
न तस्य जायते मृत्युः सत्यं सत्यं मयोदितम् ॥ 92

While he presses it, he should visualize his tongue as
joined with prana. Death does not happen for him. Truly,
I have told you the truth.

एवमभ्यासयोगेन कामदेवो द्वितीयकः ।
न क्षुधा न तृषा निद्रा नैव मूर्च्छा प्रजायते ॥ 93

By practicing thus, he becomes a second God of Love.
He gets neither hungry nor thirsty, he neither sleeps
nor swoons.

अनेनैव विधानेन योगीन्द्रोऽवनिमण्डले ।
भवेत्स्वच्छन्दचारी च सर्वापत्परिवर्जितः ॥ 94

By means of this technique, the lord of yogis becomes
able to move about the earth as he wishes and no misfor-
tunes befall him.

न तस्य पुनरावृत्तिर्मोदते स सुरैरपि ।
पुण्यपापैर्न लिप्येत होतदाचरणे सः ॥ 95

When he practices this, he is not reborn, he sports with
the gods, and he is not tainted by good and bad deeds.

चतुरशीत्यासनानि सन्ति नानाविधानि च ।
तेभ्यश्चतुष्कमादाय मयोक्तानि ब्रवीम्यहम् ॥ 96

There are eighty-four asanas of various kinds which I have
taught. Out of these I shall take four and describe them.

योनिं संपीड्य यत्नेन पादमूलेन साधकः ।
मेढ्रोपरि पादमूलं विन्यसेद्योगवित्सदा ॥ 97

The practitioner who knows Yoga should regularly and
carefully press his perineum with his heel and place the
other heel above the penis.

दृष्ट्या निरीक्ष्य भ्रूमध्यं निश्चलः संयतेन्द्रियः ।
तिष्ठेदवक्रकायश्च रहस्युद्वेगवर्जितः ॥ 98

In a lonely place and free from disturbances, he should
look between his eyebrows and remain motionless, his
senses restrained and his body straight.

एतत्सिद्धासनं ज्ञेयं सिद्धानां सिद्धिदायकम् ।
येनाभ्यासवशाच्छीघ्रं योगनिष्पत्तिमाप्नुयात् ॥ 99

This is known as Siddhasana. It grants perfection to adepts. Through practicing it, one quickly obtains the nishpatti state of Yoga.

सिद्धासनं सदा सेव्यं पवनाभ्यासिना परम् ।
येन संसारमुत्सृज्य लभते परमां गतिम् ॥ 100

Siddhasana should be used regularly by those practicing pranayama. The yogi can use it to cast off samsara and reach the ultimate destination.

नातः परतरं गुह्यमासनं विद्यते भुवि ।
येनानुध्यानमात्रेण योगी पापाद्विमुच्यते ॥ 101

This secret asana is the greatest on earth. Merely by thinking of it, the yogi is freed from sin.

उत्तानौ चरणौ कृत्वा ऊरुसंस्थौ प्रयत्नतः ।
ऊरुमध्ये तथोत्तानौ पाणी कृत्वा तु तादृशौ ॥ 102

Carefully place both feet, soles upward, on the thighs and similarly put the hands, palm upwards, on the middle of the thighs.

नासाग्रे विन्यसेदृष्टिं राजदन्तं च जिह्वया ।
उत्तम्भ्य चिबुकं वक्षे संस्थाप्य पवनं शनैः ॥ 103
यथाशक्त्या समाकृष्य पूरयेदुदरं शनैः ।
यथाशक्त्यैव पश्चात्तु रेचयेदनिरोधतः ॥ 104

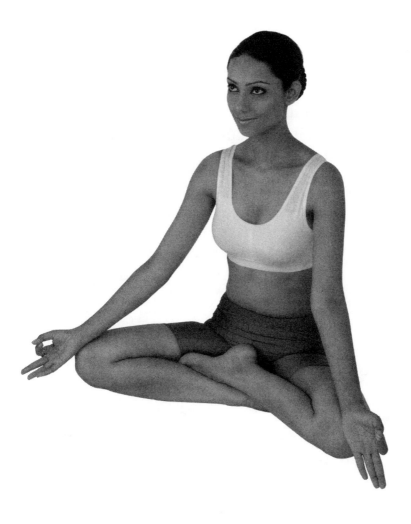

सिद्धासन – Siddhasana

Focus the gaze on the tip of the nose, push the uvula upward with the tongue, place the chin on the chest, and slowly draw in as much air as possible, gently filling up the stomach. Then exhale as much as possible, without pausing.

इदं पद्मासनं प्रोक्तं सर्वव्याधिविनाशनम् ।
दुर्लभं येन केनापि धीमता लभ्यते परम् ॥ 105

This is called Padmasana. It gets rid of all diseases and is not available to all and sundry but can be had by the wise.

अनुष्ठाने कृते प्राणः समश्चलति तत्क्षणात् ।
भवेदभ्यसने सम्यक्साधकस्य न संशयः ॥ 106

When it is performed, prana immediately flows evenly. When it is practiced repeatedly, the practitioner's prana is sure to become correct.

पद्मासनस्थितो योगी प्राणापानविधानतः ।
पूरयेत्स विमुक्तः स्यात्सत्यं सत्यं वदाम्यहम् ॥ 107

Sitting in Padmasana, the yogi should inhale while regulating prana and apana. He becomes liberated. Truly, I speak the truth.

प्रसार्य चरणद्वन्द्वं परस्परसुसंयुतम् ।
स्वपाणिभ्यां दृढं धृत्वा जानूपरि शिरो न्यसेत् ॥ 108

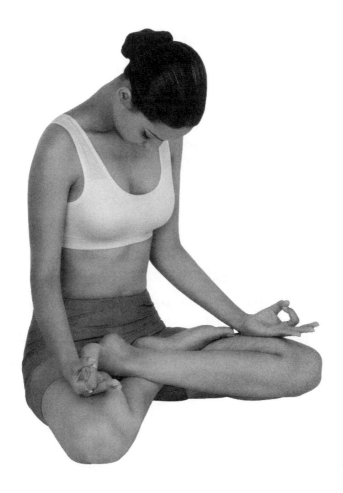

पद्मासन – Padmasana

Join both feet together and extend them. Hold them firmly with both hands and place the head on the knees.

आसनाग्र्यमिदं प्रोक्तं जठरानलदीपनम् ।
देहावसादहरणं पश्चिमोत्तानसंज्ञकम् ॥ 109

This foremost asana is said to kindle the digestive fire. It removes physical exhaustion and is called Paschimottanasana.

य एतदासनं श्रेष्ठं प्रत्यहं साधयेत्सुधीः ।
वायुः पश्चिममार्गेण तस्य संचरति ध्रुवम् ॥ 110

The breath of the wise yogi who practices this excellent asana every day is sure to travel by the rearward path.

एतदभ्यासशीलानां सर्वसिद्धिः प्रजायते ।
तस्माद्योगी प्रयत्नेन साधयेत्सिद्धिसाधकः ॥ 111

Those who practice it attain every perfection, so the yogi who wants to attain perfections should practice it assiduously.

गोपनीयं प्रयत्नेन न देयं यस्य कस्यचित् ।
येन शीघ्रं मरुत्सिद्धिर्भवेद्दुःखौघनाशिनी ॥ 112

It is to be carefully guarded and not given to all and sundry. By means of it, mastery of the wind, which destroys a host of sorrows, quickly arises.

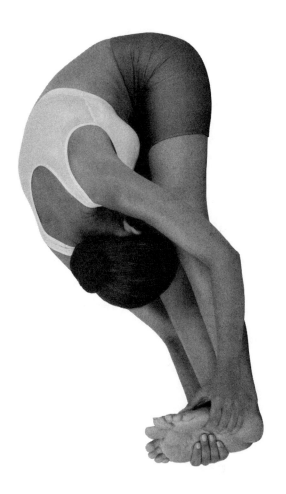

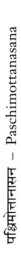

पश्चिमोत्तानासन – Paschimottanasana

जानूर्वोरन्तरे सम्यक्कृत्वा पादतले उभे ।
समकायः समासीनः स्वस्तिकं तत्प्रचक्षते ॥ 113

Put the soles of both feet directly between the thighs and
the calves and sit up straight. This is called Svastikasana.

अनेन विधिना योगी मारुतं साधयेत्सुधीः ।
देहे न क्रमते व्याधिस्तस्य वायुश्च सिध्यति ॥ 114

The wise yogi should practice pranayama using this asana.
Disease does not enter his body and he attains mastery
of the wind.

सुखासनमिदं प्रोक्तं सर्वदुःखप्रणाशनम् ।
स्वस्तिकं योगिभिर्गोप्यं स्वस्थीकरणमुत्तमम् ॥ 115

This is also called Sukhasana, the easy asana. It destroys
all suffering. Svastikasana is the best for making one
healthy and is to be kept secret by yogis."

इति श्रीशिवसंहितायां योगशास्त्रे ईश्वरपार्वतीसंवादे
तृतीयः पटलः ॥

Thus ends the third chapter in the glorious *Shiva Samhita*,
a treatise on Yoga in the form of a dialogue between the
Lord and Parvati.

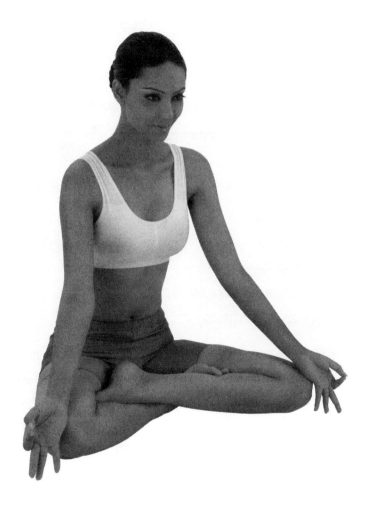

स्वस्तिकासन – Svastikasana

Chapter Four

Mudras

ईश्वर उवाच ।
अथातः संप्रवक्ष्यामि मुद्रिकायोगमुत्तमम् ।
तस्या अभ्यासमात्रेण सर्वव्याधिः प्रमुच्यते ॥ 1

The Lord said, "Now I shall teach the sublime Yoga of mudras. Just by practicing mudras the yogi is freed from all disease.

आदौ पूरकयोगेन स्वाधारे धारयेन्मनः ।
गुदमेढ्रान्तरे योनिस्तामाकुंच्य प्रवर्तयेत् ॥ 2

First fix the mind in the Adhara by means of inhalation. There is a yoni between the anus and the penis. Contract it and make it active.

ब्रह्मयोनिगतं ध्यात्वा कामं कन्दुकसंनिभम् ।
तस्योर्ध्वे तु शिखा सूक्ष्मा चिद्रूपा परमा कला ॥ 3

Meditate on the God of Love as residing in Brahma's yoni in the shape of a ball, looking like ten million suns and as cool as ten million moons.

तया सहितमात्मानमेकीभूतं विचिन्तयेत् ।
गच्छति ब्रह्ममार्गेण लिंगत्रयक्रमेण वै ॥ 4
सूर्यकोटिप्रतीकाशं चन्द्रकोटिसुशीतलम् ।
अमृतं तद्धि स्वर्गस्थं परमानन्दलक्षणम् ।
श्वेतरक्तं तेजसाढ्यं धारापातैः प्रवर्षिणम् ॥ 5

Above it is the ultimate digit, a tiny flame whose form is
consciousness. The yogi should imagine himself as having
become one with it. He goes along the way of Brahma,
progressing through the three lingas, to the nectar of
immortality which is in heaven, characterized by ultimate
bliss, pink, abounding in vital energy, and pouring forth
showers of rain.

पीत्वा कुलामृतं दिव्यं पुनरेव विशेत्कुलम् ।
पुनरेव कुलं गच्छेन्मात्रायोगेन नान्यथा ॥ 6

After drinking the divine nectar of the Kula[1] the yogi
should enter the Kula once more. He should go again to
the Kula by means of pranayama, not otherwise.

सा च प्राणसमाख्याता ह्यस्मिंस्तन्त्रे मयोदिते ।
पुनः प्रलीयते तस्यां कालाग्न्यादिशिवान्तकम् ॥ 7

In this tantra I have called her prana. That which begins
with the fire of time and ends in Shiva is absorbed in her
once more.

---

[1] In the *Shiva Samhita*, Kula means the Adhara lotus. See verse 5.88.

योनिमुद्रा परा होषा बन्धस्तस्याः प्रकीर्तितः ।
तस्यास्तु बन्धमात्रेण तन्नास्ति यन्न साधयेत् ॥ ८

This is the great Yonimudra. Its application has been
taught. Just by applying it one can do anything.

छिन्नरूपास्तु ये मन्त्राः कीलिताः स्तम्भिताश्च ये ।
दग्धाः मन्त्राः शिखाहीनाः मलिनास्तु तिरस्कृताः ॥ ९
भेदिता भ्रमसंयुक्ताः शप्ताः संमूर्छिताश्च ये ।
मन्दा बालास्तथा वृद्धाः प्रौढाः यौवनगर्विताः ।
अरिपक्षे स्थिता ये च निर्वीर्याः सत्त्ववर्जिताः ॥ १०
तथा सत्त्वेन हीनाश्च खण्डिताः शतधा कृताः ।
विधिनानेन संयुक्ताः प्रभवन्त्यचिरेण तु ।
सिद्धिमोक्षप्रदाः सर्वे गुरुणा विनियोजिताः ॥ ११

Mantras that are incomplete, pierced, paralyzed, burnt
out, blunt, dirty, reviled, broken, mistaken, cursed,
unconscious, slow, young, old, audacious, proud of
their youth, on the side of the enemy, impotent, weak,
weakened, or fragmented into a hundred pieces, soon
become powerful in conjunction with this practice.
When given by a guru, they all bestow perfections
and liberation.

यद्यदुच्चरते योगी मन्त्ररूपं शुभाशुभम् ।
तत्तसिद्धिमवाप्नोति योनिमुद्रानिबन्धनात् ॥ १२

The yogi obtains mastery of whatever he utters in the form of a mantra, auspicious or otherwise, by applying the Yonimudra.

दीक्षयित्वा विधानेन अभिषिच्य सहस्रधा ।
ततो मन्त्राधिकारार्थमेषा मुद्रा प्रकीर्तिता ॥ 13

After duly initiating him and anointing him a thousand times, this mudra is taught in order to grant the right to practice mantra.

ब्रह्महत्यासहस्राणि त्रैलोक्यमपि घातयेत् ।
नासौ लिप्यति पापेन योनिमुद्रानिबन्धनात् ॥ 14

Were he to kill a thousand Brahmins and destroy the three worlds, by applying the Yonimudra he would not be tainted by sin.

गुरुहा च सुरापी च स्तेयी गुरुतल्पगः ।
एतैः पापैर्न बध्येत योनिमुद्रानिबन्धनात् ॥ 15

By applying the Yonimudra, a man who kills his guru, drinks alcohol, steals, or sleeps with his guru's wife, is not bound by these sins.

तस्मादभ्यसनं नित्यं कर्तव्यं मोक्षकांक्षिभिः ।
अभ्यासाज्जायते सिद्धिरभ्यासान्मोक्षमाप्नुयात् ॥ 16

Therefore those who desire liberation should practice regularly. Success arises through practice. Through practice one attains liberation.

संवित्तिं लभतेऽभ्यासाद्योगोऽभ्यासात्प्रवर्तते ।
मन्त्राणां सिद्धिरभ्यासादभ्यासाद्वायुसाधनम् ॥ 17

One obtains understanding through practice. Yoga happens through practice. Mantras are mastered through practice. Mastery of the wind comes through practice.

कालवंचनमभ्यासात्तथा मृत्युंजयो भवेत् ।
वाक्सिद्धिः कामचारित्वं भवेदभ्यासयोगतः ॥ 18

One deceives time through practice and conquers death. Through practice there arise mastery of speech and the ability to go where one wants.

योनिमुद्रा परं गोप्या न देया यस्य कस्यचित् ।
सर्वथा नैव दातव्या प्राणैः कण्ठगतैरपि ॥ 19

Yonimudra is to be well guarded and not given to all and sundry. It is absolutely not to be given out, even by those at their last gasp.

अधुना कथयिष्यामि योगसिद्धिकरं परम् ।
गोपनीयं तु सिद्धानां योगं परमदुर्लभम् ॥ 20

Now I shall teach the greatest means of success in Yoga. Adepts must guard this extremely precious Yoga.

सुप्ता गुरुप्रसादेन यदा जागर्ति कुण्डली ।
तदा सर्वाणि पद्मानि भिद्यन्ते ग्रन्थयोऽपि च ॥ 21

When the sleeping Kundalini awakens through the grace of the guru, all the lotuses and knots are pierced.

तस्मात्सर्वप्रयत्नेन प्रबोधयितुमीश्वरीम् ।
ब्रह्मद्वारमुखे सुप्तां मुद्राभ्यासं समाचरेत् ॥ 22

Therefore, in order to awaken the goddess sleeping at the opening of the gateway of Brahman, the yogi should make every effort to practice mudras.

महामुद्रा महाबन्धो महावेधश्च खेचरी ।
जालन्धरो मूलबन्धो विपरीतकृतिस्तथा ॥ 23
उड्यानं चैव वज्रोली दशमं शक्तिचालनम् ।
इदं हि मुद्रादशकं मुद्राणामुत्तमोत्तमम् ॥ 24

Mahamudra, Mahabandha, Mahavedha, Khechari, Jalandhara, Mulabandha, Viparitakarani, Udyana, Vajroli, and the tenth, Shaktichalana: these ten mudras are the very best mudras.

महामुद्रां प्रवक्ष्यामि तन्त्रेऽस्मिन्मम वल्लभाम् ।
यां प्राप्य सिद्धाः संसिद्धिं कपिलादयाः पुरा गताः ॥ 25

In this tantra I shall teach you Mahamudra, which is dear to me. In the past, adepts like Kapila have attained complete perfection after receiving it.

अपसव्येन संपीड्य पादमूलेन सादरम् ।
गुरूपदेशतो योनिं गुदमेढ्रान्तरालगाम् ॥ 26

Following one's guru's instructions, carefully press the yoni in the space between the anus and the penis with the left heel.

सव्यं प्रसारितं पादं धृत्वा पाणियुगेन वै ।
नवद्वाराणि संयम्य चिबुकं हृदयोपरि ॥ 27
चित्तं चित्तपथे दत्त्वा प्रारभेद्वायुधारणम् ।
महामुद्रा भवेदेषा सर्वतन्त्रेषु गोपिता ॥ 28

Stretch out the right foot and hold it with both hands. Block the nine doors, put the chin on the chest. Place the mind in the way of the mind and start holding the breath. This is Mahamudra. It is kept secret in all the tantras.

वामांगेन समभ्यस्य दक्षांगेनाभ्यसेत्पुनः ।
प्राणायामं समं कृत्वा योगी नियतमानसः ॥ 29

After practicing on the left side of the body, the yogi, his mind restrained, should balance his pranayama and practice again on the right.

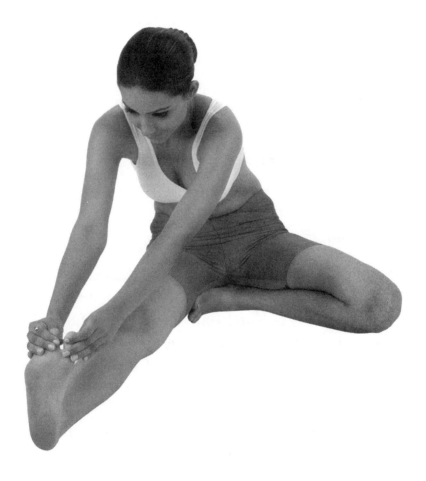

महामुद्रा – Mahamudra

मुद्रामेतां तु संप्राप्य गुरुवक्त्रात्सुशोभिताम् ।
अनेन विधिना योगी मन्दभाग्योऽपि सिध्यति ॥ 30

After receiving this glorious mudra from his guru's mouth, even an ill-starred yogi can achieve success with this technique.

सर्वासामेव नाडीनां चालनं बिन्दुधारणम् ।
जारनं तु कषायस्य पातकानां विनाशनम् ॥ 31
कुण्डलीतापनं वायोर्ब्रह्मरन्ध्रप्रवेशनम् ।
सर्वरोगोपशमनं जठराग्निविवर्धनम् ॥ 32
वपुषः कान्तिरमला जरामृत्युविनाशनम् ।
वांछितार्थफलं सौख्यमिन्द्रियाणां च मारणम् ॥ 33
एतदुक्तानि सर्वाणि योगारूढस्य योगिनः ।
भवेदभ्यासतोऽवश्यं नात्र कार्या विचारणा ॥ 34

The ability to make all the nadis flow, the steadying of bindu, the incineration of impurities, the destruction of sins, the heating of Kundalini, the insertion of the wind into the aperture of Brahman, the curing of all diseases, the increase of the digestive fire, perfect physical beauty, the destruction of old age and death, the achievement of desired goals, happiness, and the conquest of the senses: through practice, all these arise for the yogi on the path of Yoga. This is not to be doubted.

गोपनीया प्रयत्नेन मुद्रेयं सुरपूजिता ।
यां च प्राप्य भवाम्भोधेः पारं गच्छन्ति योगिनः ॥ 35

This mudra is worshipped by the gods and is to be carefully guarded. On obtaining it, yogis cross the ocean of worldly existence.

मुद्रा कामदुधा ह्येषा साधकानां मयोदिता ।
गुप्ताचारेण कर्तव्या न देया यस्य कस्यचित् ॥ 36

This mudra that I have taught grants practitioners their every desire. It is to be performed secretly and not given to all and sundry.

तस्यां प्रसारितः पादो विन्यस्य तमुरूपरि ।
गुदयोनिं समाकुंच्य कृत्वा चापानमूर्ध्वगम् ॥ 37

While in Mahamudra, place the foot that is extended upon the thigh. Contract the anus and yoni and make the apana move upwards.

योजयित्वा समानेन कृत्वा प्राणमधोमुखम् ।
बन्धयेतूर्ध्वगत्यर्थं हि प्राणापानयोः सुधी ॥ 38

Join prana with samana and make it face downwards. The wise yogi should apply this in order to make prana and apana move upwards.

कथितोऽयं महाबन्धः सिद्धिमार्गप्रदायकः ।
नाडीजालादृसव्यूहो मूर्धानं याति योगिनः ॥ 39

This Mahabandha that I have taught leads the way to perfection. All the yogi's fluids go from the network of nadis to the head.

उभाभ्यां साधयेत्पदाभ्यामेकैकं सुप्रयत्नतः ।
भवेदभ्यासतो वायुः सुषुम्णामध्यसंगतः ॥ 40

One should take great care to practice this with both feet alternately. Through practice, the wind enters the Sushumna.

अनेन वपुषः पुष्टिर्दृढबन्धोऽस्थिपञ्जरः ।
संपूर्णहृदयो योगी भवन्त्येतानि योगिनः ॥ 41

It nourishes the body, makes the skeleton strong, and fills the yogi's heart. These things arise for the yogi.

बन्धेनानेन योगीन्द्रः साधयेत्सर्वमीप्सितम् ।
अपानप्राणयोरैक्यं कृत्वा त्रिभुवनेष्वपि ॥ 42

Using this bandha, the lord of yogis unites prana and apana and accomplishes all that he desires in the three worlds.

महाबन्धस्थितो योगी कुक्षिमापूर्य वायुना ।
स्फिचौ संतापयेद्भूमिान्वेधोऽयं कीर्तितो मया ॥ 43

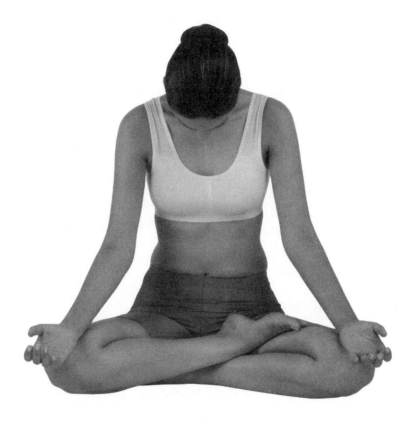

महाबन्ध – Mahabandha

While seated in Mahabandha, the wise yogi should fill
his belly with air and tap his buttocks. This is the Vedha
taught by me.

वेधेनानेन संविध्य वायुना योगिपुंगवः ।
ग्रन्थीन्सुषुम्णामार्गेण ब्रह्मरन्ध्रं भिनत्त्यसौ ॥ 44

The best of yogis, having by means of this Vedha used his
breath to pierce the knots along the Sushumna, breaks
through the aperture of Brahman.

यः करोति सदाभ्यासं महावेधं सुगोपितम् ।
वायुसिद्धिर्भवित्तस्य जरामरणनाशिनी ॥ 45

Mastery of the wind, which destroys decrepitude and
death, arises for the yogi who regularly practices the
secret Mahavedha.

चक्रमध्ये स्थिता देवाः कम्पन्ते वायुताडनात् ।
कुण्डल्यपि महामाया कैलासे सा विलीयते ॥ 46

The gods in the middle of the chakra tremble when
the wind is struck and the great goddess of illusion,
Kundalini, is absorbed into Kailasa.

महामुद्रामहाबन्धौ निष्फलौ वेधवर्जितौ ।
तस्माद्योगी प्रयत्नेन करोति त्रितयं क्रमात् ॥ 47

Without Vedha, Mahamudra and Mahabandha do not bear fruit, so the yogi should carefully practice all three in succession.

एतत्त्रयं प्रयत्नेन चतुर्वारं करोति यः ।
षण्मासाभ्यन्तरे मृत्युं जयत्येव न संशयः ॥ 48

He who carefully practices this triad four times a day is sure to conquer death within six months.

एतत्त्रयस्य माहात्म्यं सिद्धो जानाति नेतरः ।
यज्ज्ञात्वा साधकाः सर्वे सिद्धिं सम्यग्लभन्ति च ॥ 49

Only the adept understands the importance of this triad and, on realizing it, all practitioners duly achieve perfection.

गोपनीयं प्रयत्नेन साधकैः सिद्धिमीप्सुभिः ।
अन्यथा च न सिद्धिः स्यान्मुद्राणामेष निश्चयः ॥ 50

It is to be guarded carefully by practitioners desiring perfection, otherwise the mudras are certain not to be mastered.

भ्रुवोरन्तर्गतां दृष्टिं विधाय सुदृढं सुधीः ।
उपविश्यासने वज्रे नानोपद्रववर्जितः ॥ 51

The wise yogi should sit in Vajrasana and, free from any disturbances, firmly fix his gaze between the eyebrows.

लम्बिकोर्ध्वस्थिते गर्ते रसनां विपरीतगाम् ।
संयोजयेत्प्रयत्नेन सुधाकूपे विचक्षणः ॥ 52

The clever yogi should turn back his tongue and carefully insert it into the well of nectar in the hollow
above the uvula.

मुद्रैषा खेचरी प्रोक्ता भक्तानामनुरोधतः ।
सिद्धीनां जननी होषा मम प्राणाधिकप्रिया ॥ 53

I have taught this Khecharimudra out of affection for my
devotees. It brings about perfections and is more dear to
me than life.

निरन्तरकृताभ्यासात्पीयूषं प्रत्यहं पिबेत् ।
तेन विग्रहसिद्धिः स्यान्मृत्युमातंगकेसरी ॥ 54

Through regular practice, the yogi drinks nectar every
day, as a result of which perfection of the body arises, a
lion against the elephant of death.

अपवित्रः पवित्रो वा सर्वावस्थां गतोऽपि वा ।
खेचरीं कुरुते यस्तु स शुद्धो नात्र संशयः ॥ 55

Whatever condition a man may be in, pure or impure, if
he knows Khechari he is sure to be purified.

क्षणार्धं कुरुते यस्तु तीर्वा पापमहार्णवम् ।

दिव्यभोगान् च भुक्त्वैव सत्कुले स प्रजायते ॥ 56

He who practices it for half an instant crosses the ocean
of sin and enjoys divine delights before being born into
a good family.

खेचर्या मुद्रया यस्तु सुस्थितः स्यादतन्द्रितः ।
शतब्रह्मगतेनापि क्षणार्धं मन्यते हि सः ॥ 57

He who remains comfortably and without fatigue in
Khecharimudra, reckons a hundred ages of Brahma to
be half an instant.

गुरूपदेशतो मुद्रां यो वेत्ति खेचरीमिमाम् ।
नानापापरतो धीमान्स याति परमां गतिम् ॥ 58

The wise yogi, who knows this Khecharimudra from the
instruction of his guru, reaches the ultimate destination
while delighting in a multitude of sins.

स्वप्राणैः सदृशो यस्तु तस्मा अपि न दीयते ।
प्रच्छाद्यातिप्रयत्नेन मुद्रेयं सुरपूजिता ॥ 59

It is not given even to him who is as dear as one's own
life. This mudra which is worshipped by the gods is to be
guarded with great care.

बद्ध्वा गलशिराजालं हृदये चिबुकं न्यसेत् ।

बन्धो जालन्धरः प्रोक्तो देवानामपि दुर्लभः ॥ 60

Constrict the network of vessels in the neck and place the chin on the chest. This is called Jalandharabandha. It is precious even to the gods.

नाभिस्थवह्निर्जन्तूनां सहस्रकमलच्युतम् ।
पिबेत्पीयूषविसरं तदर्थं बन्धयेदिदम् ॥ 61

In living beings, the fire situated at the navel drinks the abundance of nectar pouring from the thousand-petaled lotus. That is why one should apply this bandha.

बन्धेनानेन पीयूषं स्वयं पिबति बुद्धिमान् ।
अमरत्वं च संप्राप्य मोदते भुवनत्रये ॥ 62

By applying this bandha, the wise yogi drinks the nectar himself. He becomes immortal and has fun in the three worlds.

जालन्धरो बन्ध एष सिद्धानां सिद्धिदायकः ।
अभ्यासः क्रियते नित्यं योगिना सिद्धिमिच्छता ॥ 63

This Jalandharabandha grants perfection to adepts. The yogi desirous of perfection should carry out the practice regularly.

पादमूलेन संपीड्य गुदामार्गं सुयन्त्रितम् ।

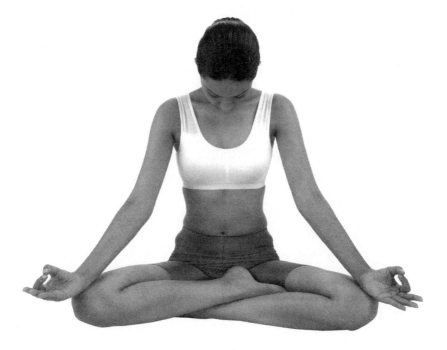

जालन्धरबन्ध & मूलबन्ध – Jalandharabandha & Mulabandha

बलादपानमाकृष्य क्रमादूर्ध्वं तु चारयेत् ॥ 64

Press the anus tightly with the heel. Forcefully pull the apana and gradually raise it.

कल्पितोऽयं मूलबन्धो जरामरणनाशनः ।
अपानप्राणयोरैक्यं प्रकरोत्यविकम्पितम् ॥ 65

This makes Mulabandha. It destroys decrepitude and death, and is sure to unite apana and prana.

बन्धेनानेन सुतरां योनिमुद्रा प्रसिध्यति ।
सिद्धायां योनिमुद्रायां किं न सिध्यति भूतले ॥ 66

By applying this bandha, Yonimudra is easily perfected. When Yonimudra is perfected, there is nothing on earth that one cannot master.

बन्धस्यास्य प्रसादेन गगने विजितानिलः ।
पद्मासनस्थितो योगी भुवमुत्सृज्य वर्तते ॥ 67

By grace of this mudra, the yogi sitting in Padmasana conquers the wind and leaves the ground to dwell in the sky.

सुगुप्ते निर्जने देशे बन्धमेनं समभ्यसेत् ।
संसारसागरं तर्त्तुं यदीच्छेद्योगिपुंगवः ॥ 68

If the best of yogis wants to cross the ocean of samsara, he should practice this mudra in a secret place free from people.

भूतले स्वशिरो दत्त्वा खे नयेच्चरणद्वयम् ।
विपरीतकृतिश्चैषा सर्वतन्त्रेषु गोपिता ॥ 69

Place the head on the ground and both feet in the air.
This Viparitakarani is kept secret in all the tantras.

एतां यः कुरुते नित्यमभ्यासाद्यामममात्रकम् ।
मृत्युं जयति योगी सः प्रलये नापि सीदति ॥ 70

From daily practice for a period of three hours, the yogi
who performs it conquers death and does not perish even
at the cosmic dissolution.

अमृतं कुरुते पानं सिद्धानां समतामियात् ।
स सेव्यः सर्वलोकानां बन्धमेनं करोति यः ॥ 71

He drinks the nectar of immortality and becomes equal
to the adepts. He who performs this bandha is to be worshipped by the whole world.

नाभेरूर्ध्वमधश्चापि तानं पश्चिममाचरेत् ।
उड्यानबन्ध एषः स्यात्सर्वदुःखौघनाशनः ॥ 72

The yogi should stretch the region above and below the
navel backwards. This is Udyanabandha. It destroys all
one's many sorrows.

उदरे पश्चिमं तानं नाभेरूर्ध्वं तु कारयेत् ।

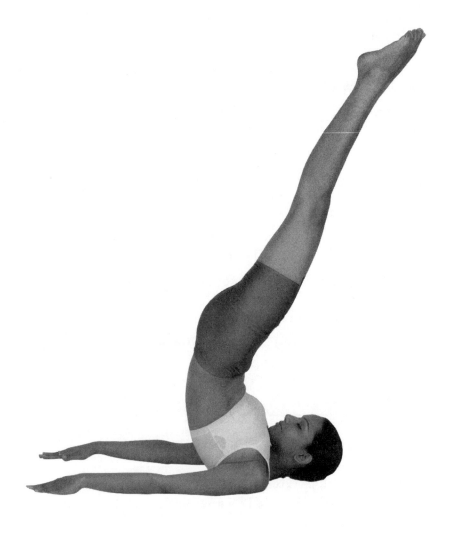

विपरीतकरणी – Viparitakarani

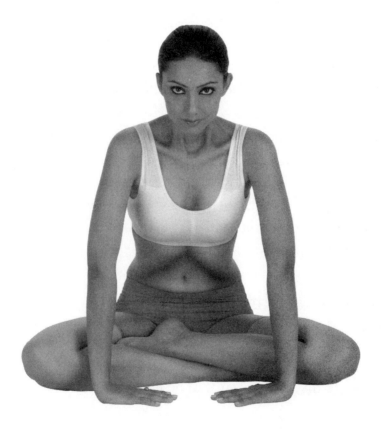

उड्डयानबन्ध – Udyanabandha

उड्यानाख्योऽत्र बन्धोऽयं मृत्युमातंगकेसरी ॥ 73

He should stretch it to behind the stomach and above the navel. In this text this bandha is called Udyana.[2] It is a lion against the elephant of death.

नित्यं यः कुरुते योगी चतुर्वारं दिने दिने ।
तस्य नाभेस्तु शुद्धिः स्यात्सिद्धो भवति मारुतः ॥ 74

The navel of the yogi who regularly performs it four times a day is purified and the wind is mastered.

षण्मासमभ्यसन्योगी मृत्युं जयति निश्चितम् ।
तस्योदराग्निर्ज्वलति रसवृद्धिश्च जायते ॥ 75

Practicing it for six months, the yogi is sure to conquer death. The fire in his stomach burns brightly and there is an increase in his vital fluids.

अनेन सुतरां सिद्धिर्विग्रहस्य प्रजायते ।
रोगाणां संक्षयश्चापि योगिनो भवति ध्रुवम् ॥ 76

The body easily becomes perfected through using it and the yogi's diseases are sure to be eliminated.

गुरोर्लब्ध्वा प्रयत्नेन साधयेत्तु विचक्षणः ।
निर्जने सुस्थिते देशे बन्धं परमदुर्लभम् ॥ 77

---

[2]This bandha is usually called Uddiyana.

The wise yogi should obtain this extremely precious bandha from a guru and practice it in a comfortable place where there are no people.

वज्रोलीं कथयिष्यामि संसारध्वान्तनाशिनीम् ।
स्वभक्तेभ्यः समासेन गुह्यादुह्यतमामपि ॥ 78

I shall teach my devotees a summary of Vajroli, the secret of all secrets, the destroyer of the darkness of samsara.

स्वेच्छया वर्तमानोऽपि योगोक्तनियमैर्विना ।
मुक्तो भवेद्गृहस्थोऽपि वज्रोल्यभ्यासयोगतः ॥ 79

Through the practice of Vajroli, even a householder living according to his desires and without the restrictions taught in Yoga can be liberated.

वज्रोल्या सह योगोऽयं भोगे भुक्तेऽपि मुक्तिदः ।
तस्मादतिप्रयत्नेन कर्तव्यो योगिभिः सदा ॥ 80

Together with Vajroli, this Yoga grants liberation even to one who indulges his senses, so it should be regularly and zealously practiced by yogis.

आदौ रजः स्त्रियो योन्या यत्नेन विधिवत्सुधीः ।
आकुंच्य लिंगनालेन स्वशरीरे प्रवेशयेत् ॥ 81

First the wise yogi should carefully and correctly draw up through his urethra the generative fluid from a woman's vagina and make it enter his body.

स्वकं बिन्दुं च संबोध्य लिंगचालनमाचरेत् ।
दैवाञ्चलति चेदूर्ध्वं निबद्धो योनिमुद्रया ॥ 82

After awakening his semen he should start to move his penis. If by chance his semen should move upwards it can be stopped with the Yonimudra.

वाममार्गेऽपि तद्बिन्दुं नीत्वा लिंगं निवारयेत् ।
क्षणमात्रं योनितोऽयं पुनश्चालनमाचरेत् ॥ 83

He should draw his semen onto the left side, remove his penis from the vagina for a moment, and then start having intercourse again.

गुरूपदेशतो योगी हुंहुंकारेण योनितः ।
अपानवायुमाकुंच्य बलादाकर्षयेद्द्रजः ॥ 84

Following his guru's instructions, the yogi should draw up his apana wind and with the sound *hum hum* forcibly extract the generative fluid from the yoni.

अनेन विधिना योगी क्षिप्रं योगस्य सिद्धये ।
गव्यभुक्कुरुते योगी गुरुपादाम्बुजपूजकः ॥ 85

In order to obtain success in Yoga quickly by means of this practice, the yogi who worships his guru's lotus feet eats the products of the cow.

बिन्दुर्विधुमयो ज्ञेयो रजः सूर्यमयस्तथा ।
उभयोर्मेलनं कार्यं स्वशरीरे प्रयत्नतः ॥ 86

Know semen to be lunar and the generative fluid to be solar. One should strive to combine them both in one's own body.

अहं बिन्दुः रजः शक्तिरुभयोर्मेलनं यदा ।
योगिनां साधनवतां भवेद्दिव्यं वपुस्तदा ॥ 87

I am semen, the goddess is the generative fluid. When both are combined, the body of the practicing yogi becomes divine.

मरणं बिन्दुपातेन जीवनं बिन्दुधारणे ।
तस्मादतिप्रयत्नेन कुरुते बिन्दुधारणम् ॥ 88

Death arises through the falling of semen, life when it is retained. Therefore one should do one's utmost to retain one's semen.

जायते म्रियते लोके बिन्दुना नात्र संशयः ।
एतज्ज्ञात्वा सदा योगी बिन्दुधारणमाचरेत् ॥ 89

One is born and dies in the world through semen. In this there is no doubt. Knowing this, the yogi should always retain his semen.

सिद्धे बिन्दौ महारत्ने किं न सिध्यति भूतले ।
यस्य प्रसादान्महिमा ममाप्येतादृशी भवेत् ॥ ९०

When the great jewel semen is mastered there is nothing on earth that cannot be mastered. Through its grace, one becomes as great as me.

बिन्दुः करोति सर्वेषां सुखं दुःखं च संस्थितः ।
संसारिणां विमूढानां जरामरणशालिनाम् ॥ ९१

Semen, depending on its state, brings about happiness and sorrow for all the deluded inhabitants of the world subject to decrepitude and death.

अयं शुभकरो योगो योगिनामुत्तमोत्तमः ।
अभ्यासात्सिद्धिमाप्नोति भोगे भुक्तेऽपि मानवः ॥ ९२

This auspicious Yoga is the best of all for yogis. Through its practice a man obtains perfection even if he indulges his senses.

सकलः साधितार्थोऽपि सिद्धो भवति भूतले ।
भुक्त्वा भोगानशेषान्वै योगेनानेन निश्चितम् ॥ ९३

Every goal that is sought after is sure to be achieved here
on earth by means of this Yoga, even after enjoying
all pleasures.

अनेन सकला सिद्धिर्योगिनां भवति ध्रुवम् ।
सुखभोगेन महता तस्मादेनं समभ्यसेत् ॥ 94

Using it, yogis are sure to attain total perfection, so one
should practice it while having lots of fun.

सहजोल्यमरोली च वज्रोल्या भेदतो भवेत् ।
येन केन प्रकारेण बिन्दुं योगी प्रसाधयेत् ॥ 95

Sahajoli and Amaroli are variations of Vajroli. The yogi
should use any and every means to master his semen.

दैवाञ्चलति चेद्गे मेलनं चन्द्रसूर्ययोः ।
अमरोलीरियं प्रोक्ता लिङ्गनालेन शोषयेत् ॥ 96

If his semen should accidentally enter the vagina, then the
resultant combination of the moon and the sun is called
Amaroli, and he should suck it up through his urethra.

गतं बिन्दुं स्वकं योगी बन्धयेद्योनिमुद्रया ।
सहजोलीरियं प्रोक्ता सर्वतन्त्रेषु गोपिता ॥ 97

When his semen moves, the yogi should restrain it with
Yonimudra. This is called Sahajoli and is kept secret in
all the tantras.

संज्ञाभेदाङ्गवेद्रेदः कार्ये तुल्या गतिर्यया ।
तस्मात्सर्वप्रयत्नेन साध्यते योगिभिः सदा ॥ 98

The difference is due to a difference in name. In practice
it has the same result. Therefore yogis always make every
effort to master it.

अयं योगो मया प्रोक्तो भक्तानां स्नेहतः परम् ।
गोपनीयः प्रयत्नेन न देयो यस्य कस्यचित् ॥ 99

I have taught this Yoga out of great affection for my
devotees. It is to be guarded well and not given to all
and sundry.

एतद्गुह्यतमं गुह्यं न भूतं न भविष्यति ।
तस्मादतिप्रयत्नेन गोपनीयं सदा बुधैः ॥ 100

There has never been a secret as secret as this, nor
will there ever be, so the wise should always guard it
very carefully.

स्वमूत्रोत्सर्गकाले यो बलादाकृष्य वायुना ।
स्तोकं स्तोकं त्यजेन्मूत्रमूर्ध्वमाकृष्य तत्पुनः ॥ 101
गुरूपदिष्टमार्गेण प्रत्यहं यः समाचरेत् ।
बिन्दुसिद्धिर्भवेत्तस्य महासिद्धिप्रदायिका ॥ 102

For the yogi who uses his wind to force back his urine
when urinating and then releases it bit by bit while
holding it up, and who practices every day according to

the way taught by his guru, there arises the mastery of semen, which grants great success.

षण्मासमभ्यसेद्यो वै प्रत्यहं गुरुशिक्षया ।
शतांगनोपभोगेऽपि न बिन्दुस्तस्य नश्यति ॥ 103

The semen of the yogi who practices daily for six months according to his guru's instructions is never lost, even if he enjoys a hundred women.

सिद्धे बिन्दौ महारत्ने किं न सिध्यति भूतले ।
ईशत्वं यत्प्रसादेन ममापि सुलभं भवेत् ॥ 104

When the great jewel semen is mastered, there is nothing on earth that cannot be mastered. By its grace, even my majesty is easily obtained.

आधारकमले सुप्तां चालयेत्कुण्डलीं दृढम् ।
अपानवायुमारुह्य बलादाकृष्य बुद्धिमान् ॥ 105

The wise yogi should thoroughly agitate Kundalini, who is asleep in the Adhara lotus, and force her upwards by raising the apana wind.

शक्तिचालनमेनं हि प्रत्यहं यः समाचरेत् ।
आयुर्वृद्धिर्भवेत्तस्य रोगाणां च विनाशनम् ॥ 106

The lifespan of the yogi who practices this Shaktichalana every day is extended and his diseases are destroyed.

विहाय निद्रां भुजगी स्वयमूर्ध्वं व्रजेत्खलु ।
तस्मादभ्यसनं कार्यं योगिना सिद्धिमिच्छता ॥ 107

Shaking off sleep, the serpent rises up automatically,
so the yogi desirous of perfection should carry out
the practice.

यः करोति सदाभ्यासं शक्तिचालनमुत्तमम् ।
येन विग्रहसिद्धिः स्यादणिमादिगुणप्रदा ॥ 108
गुरूपदेशविधिना तस्य मृत्युभयं कुतः ।
मुहूर्तद्वयपर्यन्तं विधिना शक्तिचालनम् ॥ 109
यः करोति प्रयत्नेन तस्य सिद्धिर्न दूरतः ।
मुक्तासनेन कर्तव्यं योगिभिः शक्तिचालनम् ॥ 110

For the yogi who constantly practices according to his
guru's instructions the sublime Shaktichalana which
brings about perfection of the body and bestows the
powers of becoming infinitesimal and so forth, there is
no fear of death. For the yogi who takes pains to practice
Shaktichalana according to the rules for two muhurtas,[3]
perfection is near at hand. Yogis should practice Shaktichalana in Muktasana.

एतत्तु मुद्रादशकं न भूतं न भविष्यति ।
एकैकाभ्यसने सिद्धे सिद्धिर्भवति नान्यथा ॥ 111

---

[3]A muhurta is forty-eight minutes.

There never were ten mudras like these nor will there ever be. Perfection arises when the practice of each one is mastered. It does not happen otherwise."

इति श्रीशिवसंहितायां योगशास्त्रे ईश्वरपार्वतीसंवादे चतुर्थः पटलः ॥

Thus ends the fourth chapter in the glorious *Shiva Samhita*, a treatise on Yoga in the form of a dialogue between the Lord and Parvati.

Chapter Five

Meditation

श्रीदेव्युवाच ।
ब्रूहि मे वाक्यमीशान परमार्थधियं प्रति ।
ये विघ्नाः सन्ति लोकानां चेन्मयि प्रेम शंकर ॥ 1

The glorious Goddess said, "If you love me, O Lord Shankara, tell me what obstacles to understanding the Ultimate Reality are faced by people."

ईश्वर उवाच ।
शृणु देवि प्रवक्ष्यामि यथा विघ्नाः स्थिताः सदा ।
मुक्तिं प्रति नराणां च भोगः परमबाधकः ॥ 2

The Lord said, "Listen, O Goddess! I shall tell you the obstacles that are always present. The greatest hindrance to liberation for people is enjoyment.

नारी शय्यासनं वस्त्रं धनमास्यविचुम्बनम् ।
ताम्बूलभक्ष्यं पानानि राज्यशौर्यविभूतयः ॥ 3
हेम रूप्यं तथा ताम्रं रत्नान्यगुरुधेनवः ।

पाण्डित्यं वेदशास्त्राणि नृत्यं गीतं विभूषणम् ॥ ४
वंशीवीणामृदंगाश्र गजेन्द्रोच्चाश्ववाहनम् ।
दारापत्यानि विषया विघ्ना एते प्रकीर्तिताः ॥ ५

Women, lying about on beds, clothes, money, kissing on
the mouth, chewing pan,[1] drinking, kingship, heroism,
wealth, gold, silver, copper, gems, fragrant aloe wood,
cows, scholarship, Vedic treatises, dancing, singing,
jewelry, flutes, lutes, drums, riding on elephants and tall
horses, wives, children, and sensuality: these are said
to be obstacles.

भोगरूपा इमे विघ्ना धर्मरूपानिमान् शृणु ।
स्नानं पूजा तिथिर्होमस्तथा शौचमयी स्थितिः ॥ ६
व्रतोपवासनियमा मौनमिन्द्रियनिग्रहः ।
ध्येयो ध्यानं तथा मन्त्रो दानं ख्यातिर्दिशासु च ॥ ७
वापीकूपतडागादिप्रासादारामकल्पना ।
यज्ञं चन्द्रायणं कृच्छ्रं तीर्थानि विविधानि च ॥ ८

These obstacles take the form of enjoyment. Now hear
about the following, which take the form of religion:
ritual bathing, worship, lunar days, making fire offerings,
propriety with regard to purity, vows, fasting, rules,
silence, restraining the senses, the object of meditation,
meditation, mantra, charity, widespread fame; the building
of pools, wells, tanks, other water sources, mansions, and

---

[1]Pan is a mixture of spices, sweets, and betel nuts.

pleasure gardens; sacrifice, the Chandrayana penance,[2] and the various pilgrimage sites.

दृश्यन्ते च इमे विघ्ना धर्मरूपेण संस्थिताः ।
येन विघ्नं भवेज्ज्ञानं कथयामि वरानने ॥ ९

These obstacles are met with in the form of religion. I shall now tell you how knowledge can become an obstacle, O beautiful one.

गोमुखाद्यासनं कृत्वा धौत्या प्रक्षालनं च तत् ।
नाडीसंचारविज्ञानं प्रत्याहारनिरोधनम् ॥ १०
कुक्षिसंचालनं क्षीरप्रवेश इन्द्रियाध्वना ।
नाडीकर्मणि कस्यापि भोजनं श्रूयतां मम ।
इत्येताः कथिता विघ्ना ज्ञानरूपे व्यवस्थिताः ॥ ११

Practicing Gomukha and other asanas after cleansing oneself internally by means of Dhauti, the science of the paths of the nadis, restraint by means of pratyahara, moving the belly from side to side, inserting milk into the urethra, eating anything according to the operations of the nadis: these are said to be the obstacles which take the form of knowledge.[3]

---

[2]The Chandrayana penance is a month-long fast beginning on the day of the full moon, on which fifteen mouthfuls of food are eaten. Each day, one less mouthful is taken until the dark of the moon, when nothing is eaten. Then one more mouthful is eaten each day, leading up to fifteen mouthfuls again on the full moon.

[3]All the manuscripts have three verses after 5.11 which are clearly a later addition to the text and very corrupt. I have omitted them.

मन्त्रयोगो हठश्चैव लययोगस्तृतीयकः ।
चतुर्थो राजयोगः स्यात्स द्विधाभाववर्जितः ॥ 12

There is Mantra Yoga and Hatha Yoga. Laya Yoga is the third. The fourth is Raja Yoga. It is free from duality.

चतुर्धा साधको ज्ञेयो मृदुमध्याधिमात्रकः ।
अधिमात्रतमः श्रेष्ठो भवाब्धिलंघनक्षमः ॥ 13

Know aspirants to be of four kinds: weak, middling, good, and outstanding. The latter is the best and can jump across the ocean of existence.

मन्दोत्साही सुसंमूढो व्याधिस्थो गुरुदूषकः ।
लोभी पापमतिश्चैव बह्वाशी वनिताश्रयः ॥ 14
चपलः कातरो रोगी पराधीनोऽतिनिष्ठुरः ।
मन्दाचारो मन्दवीर्यो ज्ञातव्यो मृदुमानवः ॥ 15

Lazy, very ignorant, sickly, offensive to his guru, greedy, evil-minded, gluttonous, lecherous, fickle, cowardly, diseased, servile, nasty, badly behaved, and feeble: the weak man is to be known thus.

द्वादशाब्दे भवेत्सिद्धिरेतस्य यत्नतः परम् ।
मन्त्रयोगाधिकारी स ज्ञातव्यो गुरुणा ध्रुवम् ॥ 16

He attains perfection after twelve years of striving. A guru should certainly consider him to be entitled to practice Mantra Yoga.

समदृष्टिः क्षमायुक्तः पुण्याकांक्षी प्रियंवदः ।
नातिप्रौढो भवान्मूढः समवीर्यबलान्वितः ॥ 17
समबुद्धिः समाभ्यासः समकायश्च सामया ।
मध्यस्थो योगमार्गेषु यथा मध्यवयोगताः ॥ 18

He who is objective, patient, desirous of merit, affable, not
too impetuous, confused by worldly existence, of normal
valor and strength, level headed, of average diligence, and
straight backed is middling on the paths of Yoga, like
those who have reached middle age.

मध्योत्साही मध्यरोगी ज्ञातव्यो मध्यविक्रमः ।
वर्षैरष्टभिरेतेषां योगावस्था प्रसिद्ध्यति ॥ 19

He should be known to be of middling keenness,
middling health, and middling valor. For these aspirants,
Yoga becomes established in eight years.

मध्यपुण्यगतो मध्य तेनैते मध्यविक्रमः ।
मध्यस्थः सर्वकार्येषु स मध्यः स्यान्न संशयः ।
एतज्ज्ञात्वैव गुरुभिर्दीयते युक्तितो लयः ॥ 20

He who is of middling merit and middling valor and
who is fair in all he does is assuredly a middling aspirant.
Recognizing this, gurus should decide to give him
Laya Yoga.

स्थिरबुद्धिर्लये युक्तः स्वाधीनो वीर्यवानपि ।

महाशयो दयायुक्तः क्षमवान्सत्त्ववानपि ॥ 21
शूरो वयःस्थः श्रद्धावान् गुरुपादाब्जपूजकः ।
योगाभ्यासरतश्चैव ज्ञातव्यश्चाधिमात्रकः ॥ 22

Determined, experienced in laya, self-reliant, strong,
high-minded, compassionate, forgiving, resolute, brave,
in the prime of life, faithful, worshipful of his guru's
lotus feet, and devoted to the practice of Yoga: the good
aspirant is to be known thus.

एतस्य सिद्धिः षड्वर्षैर्भवेदभ्यासयोगतः ।
एतस्मै दीयते धीरैः हठयोगश्च साञ्जतः ॥ 23

He can achieve perfection in six years by means of
his practice. Wise teachers give him Hatha Yoga
in its entirety.

महावीर्यान्वितोत्साही मनोज्ञः शौर्यवानपि ।
शास्त्रज्ञोऽभ्यासशीलश्च निर्मोहश्च निराकुलः ॥ 24
नवयौवनसंपन्नो मिताहारी जितेन्द्रियः ।
निर्भयश्च शुचिर्दक्षो दाता सर्वजनाश्रयः ॥ 25
अविकारी स्थिरो धीमान्यथेच्छावस्थितः क्षमी ।
सुशीलो धर्मचारी च गुप्तचेष्टः प्रियंवदः ॥ 26
शास्त्रविश्वाससम्पन्नो देवतागुरुपूजकः ।
जनसंगविरक्तश्च महाव्याधिविवर्जितः ।
अधिमात्रव्रतज्ञश्च सर्वयोगस्य साधकः ॥ 27

Endowed with great strength, energetic, charming, intrepid, learned, diligent, clearheaded, calm, in the bloom of youth, restrained in his diet, his senses subjugated, fearless, pure, talented, generous, a refuge for all, stable, steadfast, wise, content, patient, good-natured, dutiful, discreet, agreeable, having faith in the sacred texts, worshipful of gods and teachers, averse to company, free from serious illness, and experienced in the observances of the good aspirant: thus is the practitioner of all Yogas.

त्रिभिः संवत्सरैः सिद्धिरेतस्य स्यान्न संशयः ।
सर्वयोगाधिकारी स नात्र कार्या विचारणा ॥ 28

He is sure to achieve perfection in three years. He is entitled to practice all Yogas. In this there is no doubt.

प्रतीकोपासना कार्या दृष्टादृष्टफलप्रदा ।
पुनाति दर्शनादेव नात्र कार्या विचारणा ॥ 29

The yogi should practice worship of the image, which gives the reward of knowledge of present and future lives. It purifies merely by being seen. In this there is no doubt.

गाढातपे स्वप्रतिबिम्ब ईश्वरं निरीक्ष्य विस्फारितलोचनद्वयम् ।
यदा नभः पश्यति स्वप्रतीकं नभोंगणे तत्क्षणमेव पश्यति ॥ 30

When in bright sunshine a man gazes wide-eyed at the Lord in his shadow and then looks into the sky, he sees at that very moment an image of himself in the firmament.

प्रत्यहं प्रेक्षते यो वै स्वप्रतीकं नभोंगणे ।
आयुर्बुद्धिर्भवित्तस्य न मृत्युः स्यात्कदाचन ॥ 31

He who looks at his own image in the firmament every
day becomes long-lived and wise. He can never die.

यदा पश्यति संपूर्णं स्वप्रतीकं नभोंगणे ।
तदा जयः समायाति वायुं निर्जित्य तं चरेत् ॥ 32

When he sees a complete image of himself in the
firmament, he is victorious, conquers the air, and travels
through it.

यः करोति सदाभ्यासं चात्मानं विन्दते परम् ।
पूर्णनन्दैकपुरुषं स्वप्रतीकप्रसादतः ॥ 33

He who regularly carries out this practice discovers the
higher self, the one completely blissful supreme spirit,
through the grace of his own image.

यात्राकाले विवाहे च शुभे कर्मणि संकटे ।
पापक्षये पुण्यवृद्धौ प्रतीकोपासनां चरेत् ॥ 34

When the yogi is on pilgrimage, getting married,
engaged in an auspicious activity, in trouble, losing sins,
or gaining merit, he should worship his image.

निरन्तरकृताभ्यासादन्तरे पश्यति ध्रुवम् ।

तदा मुक्तिमवाप्नोति योगी नियतमानसः ॥ 35

Through regular practice he is sure to see it internally.
Then the yogi whose mind is controlled achieves liberation.

अङ्गुष्ठाभ्यामुभे श्रोत्रे तर्जनीभ्यां विलोचने ।
नासारन्ध्रे च मध्याभ्यामनामाभ्यां मुखं दृढम् ॥ 36
निरुध्य मारुतं योगी यदैवं कुरुते भृशम् ।
तदा तत्क्षणमात्मानं ज्योतीरूपं स पश्यति ॥ 37

When the yogi restrains the wind by tightly closing his
ears with his thumbs, his eyes with his index fingers,
his nostrils with his middle fingers, and his mouth with
his ring fingers, and intently carries out this practice,
then he immediately sees himself in the form of light.

तत्तेजो दृश्यते येन क्षणमात्रं निराकुलम् ।
सर्वपापविनिर्मुक्तः स याति परमां गतिम् ॥ 38

He who clearly sees that light for just an instant is freed
from all sins and goes to the ultimate destination.

निरन्तरकृताभ्यासाद्योगी विगतकल्मषः ।
सर्वं देहादि विस्मृत्य तद्भिन्नस्तु स्वयं भवेत् ॥ 39

Through regular practice the yogi is freed from sin,
forgets his body and everything else, and automatically
becomes separate from them.

यः करोति सदाभ्यासं गुप्ताचारेण मानवः ।
स वै ब्रह्मणि लीनः स्यात्पापकर्मरतो यदि ॥ 40

The yogi who practices it regularly in secret becomes
absorbed in Brahman even if he is intent on sinful acts.

गोपनीयः प्रयत्नेन सद्यःप्रत्ययकारकः ।
निर्वाणदायको लोके योगोऽयं मम वल्लभः ॥ 41

This Yoga is to be carefully guarded. It quickly proves
itself, bestows nirvana in this life, and is dear to me.

नादः संजायते तस्य क्रमेणाभ्यासतश्च वै ।
मत्तभृंगावलीवीणासदृशः प्रथमो ध्वनिः ॥ 42

And moreover, through its practice nada gradually
arises. The first sound is like that of a line of drunken
bees or a lute.

एवमभ्यासतः पश्चात्संसारध्वान्तनाशनः ।
घण्टारवसमः पश्चाद् ध्वनिर्मेघरवोपमः ॥ 43

After practicing thus there is a sound which is like the
ringing of a bell and destroys the darkness of samsara.
Then there is a sound like thunder.

ध्वनौ तस्मिन्मनो दत्त्वा यदा तिष्ठति निर्भरः ।
तदा संजायते सिद्धिर्लयस्य मम वल्लभा ॥ 44

When the yogi concentrates on that sound and remains deeply immersed in it, there arises success in laya, which is dear to me.

तत्र नादे यदा चित्तं रमते योगिनो भृशम् ।
विस्मृत्य सकलं बाह्यं नादेन सह शाम्यति ॥ 45

When the mind of the yogi is completely at rest in that nada, he forgets everything outside him and finds peace together with the nada.

एतदभ्यासयोगेन जित्वा सम्यग्गुणान्बहून् ।
सर्वारम्भपरित्यागी चिदाकाशे विलीयते ॥ 46

When by using this practice the yogi duly overcomes the many attributes, he gives up all activity and is absorbed into the ether of consciousness.

नासनं सिद्धसदृशं न कुम्भसदृशं बलम् ।
न खेचरीसमा मुद्रा न नादसदृशो लयः ॥ 47

There is no asana like Siddha, no force like breath retention, no mudra like Khechari, and no laya like nada.

इदानीं कथयिष्यामि मुक्तस्यानुभवं परम् ।
यज्ज्ञात्वा लभते मुक्तिं पापयुक्तोऽपि साधकः ॥ 48

Now I shall describe the great experience of the liberated man, on knowing which even the sinful aspirant attains liberation.

समभ्यर्च्येश्वरं सम्यक् तत्पार्श्वे योगमुत्तमम् ।
गृह्णीयात्सुस्थितो भूत्वा गुरुं संतोष्य बुद्धिमान् ॥ ४९

After duly worshiping the Lord, the wise yogi should make himself comfortable, propitiate his guru and, sitting at his side, receive the highest Yoga.

जीवादि सकलं वस्तु दत्त्वा योगविदं गुरुम् ।
संतोष्यातिप्रयत्नेन योगोऽयं गृह्यते बुधैः ॥ ५०

The wise obtain this Yoga after giving their lives and everything else they own to a guru who knows Yoga, and by making great efforts to please him.

विप्रान्संतोष्य मेधावी नानामंगलसंयुतः ।
ममालये शुचिर्भूत्वा प्रगृह्णीयाच्छुभात्मकम् ॥ ५१

After propitiating Brahmins, the wise man should receive this auspicious Yoga inside a temple of mine while attended by various lucky signs and in a state of purity.

संन्यस्यानेन विधिना प्राक्तनं विग्रहादिकम् ।
भूत्वा दिव्यवपुर्योगी गृह्णीयादूह्यमाणकम् ॥ ५२

Having used this method to cast off his old body and so forth and to receive a divine body, the yogi should do what I am about to describe.

पद्मासनस्थितो योगी जनसंगविवर्जितः ।
विज्ञाननाडीद्वितयमंगुलीभ्यां निरोधयेत् ॥ 53

Seated in Padmasana and away from human company, he should block the two vijñana nadis with his fingers.

सिद्धिस्तदाविर्भवति सुखरूपी निरञ्जनः ।
तस्मिन्परिश्रमः कार्यो येन सिद्धो भवेत्खलु ॥ 54

Perfection then manifests itself, blissful and pure. One can become an adept by means of this, so great effort should be put into it.

यः करोति सदाभ्यासं तस्य सिद्धिर्न दूरतः ।
वायुसिद्धिर्भवेत्तस्य क्रमात्पुंसो न संशयः ॥ 55

Success is not far off for the man who practices it regularly. He is sure to gradually attain mastery of the air.

सकृद्यः कुरुते योगी पापौघं नाशयेद् ध्रुवम् ।
तस्य स्यान्मध्यमे वायुप्रवेशो नात्र संशयः ॥ 56

The yogi who does it once is sure to get rid of all his sins. His wind is sure to go into the middle.

एतदभ्यासशीलो यः स योगी देवपूजितः ।
अणिमादिगुणान् लब्ध्वा विचरेद्भुवनत्रये ॥ 57

The yogi who practices it regularly is worshipped by the
gods, obtains the powers of becoming infinitesimal and
so forth, and wanders freely about the three worlds.

यस्य स्यान्निश्चलोऽभ्यासस्तद्भ्वेत्तस्य विग्रहे ।
तिष्ठेदात्मनि मेधावी स पुनः क्रीडते भृशम् ॥ 58

This occurs in the body of him whose practice is
unswerving. The wise man abides in himself; moreover,
he has a lot of fun.

एतद्योगं परं गोप्यं न देयं यस्य कस्यचित् ।
स्वप्राणैस्तु समो यस्तु तमेव कथ्यते ध्रुवम् ॥ 59

This great Yoga is to be kept secret and not given to all
and sundry. It must only be told to him who is like
one's own lifebreath.

योगी पद्मासने तिष्ठेत्कण्ठकूपे यदा स्मरन् ।
जिह्वां कृत्वा तालुमूले क्षुत्पिपासा निवर्तते ॥ 60

When the yogi sits in Padmasana, concentrates on his
Adam's apple, and puts his tongue at the base of his palate,
he feels neither hunger nor thirst.

कण्ठकूपादधः स्थाने कूर्मनाड्यस्ति शोभना ।
तस्मिन्योगी मनः दत्त्वा चित्तस्थैर्यं लभेद् भृशम् ॥ 61

In the place below the Adam's apple is the lovely Kurma nadi. When the yogi concentrates on it, his mind becomes completely still.

शिरःकपाले रुद्राक्षं विवरं चिन्तयेद्यदा ।
तदा ज्योतिःप्रकाशः स्याद्विद्द्युत्पुञ्जसमप्रभः ॥ 62

When the yogi visualizes the eye of Shiva as an aperture in his skull, then there arises a shining light as brilliant as a ball of lightning.

एतच्चिन्तनमात्रेण पापानां संक्षयो भवेत् ।
दुराचारोऽपि पुरुषो लभते परमं पदम् ॥ 63

Merely by visualizing it, sins are destroyed. Even a wicked man attains the ultimate state.

अहर्निशं यदा चिन्तां तत्करोति विचक्षणः ।
सिद्धानां दर्शनं तस्य भाषणं च भवेद् ध्रुवम् ॥ 64

Then, when the wise man continually performs this visualization, he is sure to see and speak with the adepts.

तिष्ठन्भुञ्जन्स्वपन्गच्छन् ध्यायेच्छून्यमहर्निशम् ।
तदाकाशमयो योगी चिदाकाशे विलीयते ॥ 65

If the yogi meditates on emptiness day and night—while standing still, moving, sleeping, and eating—he becomes ethereal and is absorbed in the ether of consciousness.

एतद्ध्यानं सदा कार्यं योगिना सिद्धिमिच्छता ।
निरन्तरकृताभ्यासान्मम तुल्यो भवेद् ध्रुवम् ॥ 66

This meditation should be done regularly by the yogi desirous of perfection. Through constant practice, he is sure to become my equal.

एतद्ध्यानबलाद्योगी सर्वेषां वल्लभो भवेत् ।
सर्वभूतजयं कृत्वा निराशीरपरिग्रहः ॥ 67

By the power of this meditation the yogi becomes dear to everyone. After conquering all the elements, he is free from desire and acquisitiveness.

नासाग्रं येन दृश्यते पद्मासनगतेन वै ।
मनसो मरणं तस्य खेचरत्वं प्रसिद्ध्यति ॥ 68

When the yogi sits in Padmasana and looks at the tip of his nose, his mind dies and he successfully becomes an ethereal being.

ज्योतिः पश्यति योगीन्द्रः शुद्धं शुद्धाचलोपमम् ।
तत्राभ्यासबलेनैव स्वयं तद्द्रष्टको भवेत् ॥ 69

The lord of yogis sees a bright light like a white mountain. Through the power of practicing on it, he himself becomes its guardian.

उत्तानशयनो भूमौ सुप्त्वा ध्यायेन्निरन्तरम् ।
सद्यःश्रमविनाशाय स्वयं योगी विचक्षणः ॥ 70

To remove his fatigue quickly, the wise yogi should lie on his back on the ground and meditate without pause on that light.

शिरःपाश्चात्यभागस्य ध्याने मृत्युंजयो भवेत् ।
भ्रूमध्यदृष्टिमात्रेण ह्यपरः परिकीर्तितः ॥ 71

When the rear part of the head is meditated upon, death is conquered. The unrivaled reward produced merely by looking between the eyebrows has been taught.

चतुर्विधस्य चान्नस्य रसस्त्रेधा विभज्यते ।
तत्र सारतमो भागो लिंगदेहस्य पोषकः ॥ 72

The chyle produced from the four types of food[4] is divided into three types. Of those, the most essential part nourishes the subtle body.

सप्तधातुमयं पिण्डमेकः पुष्णाति मध्यगः ।

---

[4]Food is divided into four types according to whether it is chewed, drunk, licked, or sucked.

यति विण्मूत्ररूपेण तृतीयोंऽशस्तनोर्बहिः ॥ 73

The next one nourishes the physical body, which is made of seven constituents. The third leaves the body in the form of urine and feces.

आद्यभागं द्वयं नाड्यः प्रोक्तास्ताः सकला अपि ।
प्रेषयन्ति वपुर्वायुमापादतलमस्तकम् ॥ 74

The lower two are said to be nadis, and all nadis propel wind about the body from the soles of the feet to the head.

नाडीभिराभिः सर्वाभिर्वायुः संचरते यदा ।
तदैवान्नरसो देहे साम्येनेह प्रवर्तते ॥ 75

Only when the wind moves through all these nadis is the chyle in equilibrium here in the body.

चतुर्दशानां तत्रेह व्यापारे मुख्यता मता ।
ताः समग्रा न हीनास्ताः प्राणसंचारनाडिकाः ॥ 76

Fourteen of the nadis are taught to be preeminent on account of their functions in the body. Those movers of prana are complete and not deficient.

गुदाद्द्व्यंगुलतश्चोर्ध्वं मेढ्रैकांगुलतस्त्वधः ।
एकं चास्ति समं कन्दं समन्ताच्चतुरंगुलम् ॥ 77

Two fingers above the anus and one finger below the penis is a single flat bulb four fingers across.

पश्चिमाभिमुखी योनिर्गुदमेढ्रान्तरालगा ।
तत्र कन्दं समाख्यातं तत्रास्ते कुण्डली सदा ॥ 78

Facing backwards in the space between the anus and the penis is a yoni. The bulb is said to be there. Kundalini resides there at all times.

संवेष्ट्य सकलनाडीः सार्धत्रिकुटिलाकृतिः ।
मुखे निवेश्य सा पुच्छं सुषुम्णाविवरे स्थिता ॥ 79

She is found at the opening of Sushumna. She encircles all the nadis, is coiled three and one-half times, and has inserted her tail into her mouth.

सुप्तनागोपमा ह्येषा स्फुरन्ती प्रभया स्वया ।
अहिवत्सन्धिसंस्थाना वाग्देवी बीजसंज्ञिका ॥ 80

She is like a sleeping serpent and sparkles with her own light. Made of links like a snake, she is the goddess of speech and is called bija.[5]

ज्ञेया शक्तिरियं विष्णोर्निर्मला स्वर्णभास्वरा ।
सत्त्वं रजस्तमश्चेति गुणत्रयविकस्वरा ॥ 81

---

[5] A bija, literally "seed," is a seed syllable, i.e., a monosyllabic mantra.

Know her to be the Shakti of Vishnu, spotless and brilliantly golden. She is made to expand by the three gunas: sattva, rajas, and tamas.

तत्र बन्धूकपुष्पाभं कामबीजं प्रकीर्तितम् ।
कलहंसप्रयोगेन प्रयुक्ताक्षररूपिणम् ॥ 82

The seed syllable of Kama is said to be there, looking like a bandhuka flower. With the addition of kalahamsa it takes the form of the syllable that is used.

सुषुम्णायां च संश्लिष्य बीजं तत्र वरं स्थितम् ।
शरच्चन्द्रनिभं तेजस्त्रयमेतत्पुरःस्थितम् ॥ 83

Clinging tightly to Sushumna, the precious bija is found there, a light resembling the autumn moon. This is the foremost triad.[6]

सूर्यकोटिप्रतीकाशं चन्द्रकोटिसुशीतलम् ।
एतत्त्रयं मिलित्वैव देवी त्रिपुरभैरवी ॥ 84

As bright as ten million suns and as cool as ten million moons, when this triad comes together it makes the goddess Tripurabhairavi.

बीजसंज्ञं परं तेजस्तदेव परिकीर्तितम् ।

---

[6] The members of this triad are not clear, but are perhaps the three syllables bija, kamabija, and kalahamsa.

क्रियाविज्ञानशक्तिभ्यां युतं यत्परितो भ्रमत् ॥ 85

Only that great light is said to be called the bija. Joined with the action and consciousness shaktis, it wanders all around.

उत्तिष्ठद्विसतन्त्वाभं सूक्ष्मं शोणशिखायुतम् ।
योनिस्थं तत्परं तेजः स्वयम्भूलिंगसंस्थितम् ॥ 86

That great light looks like an upright lotus fiber, is subtle, joined with a red flame, and found at the yoni and the self-born linga.

आधारपद्ममेतद्धि योनिर्यस्यास्ति कन्दतः ।
परिस्फुरद्वादिसान्तचतुर्वर्णं चतुर्दलम् ॥ 87

The latter is the Adhara lotus, at the bulb of which is a yoni. It is brilliant, contains the four syllables starting with *va* and ending in *sa*,[7] and has four petals.

कुलाभिधं सुवर्णाभं स्वयम्भूलिंगसंज्ञितम् ।
द्विरण्डो यत्र सिद्धोऽस्ति डाकिनी यत्र देवता ॥ 88

It is called Kula, is golden, and is known as the self-born linga. In it are the adept Dviranda and the goddess Dakini.

तत्पद्ममध्यगा योनिस्तत्र कुण्डलिनी स्थिता ।

---

[7]The four syllables starting with *va* and ending in *sa* are *va*, *śa*, *ṣa*, and *sa*.

तस्या ऊर्ध्वे स्फुरत्तेजः कामबीजं भ्रमन्मतम् ॥ 89

Within that lotus is the yoni where Kundalini is found. Above her is a sparkling light taught to be the wandering bija of Kama.

यः करोति सदा ध्यानं मूलाधारे विचक्षणः ।
तस्य स्याद्दार्दुरीसिद्धिर्भूमित्यागः क्रमेण वै ॥ 90

The wise man who regularly meditates upon the Muladhara gradually attains Darduri siddhi, the ability to leave the ground like a frog.

वपुषः कान्तिरुत्कृष्टा जठराग्निविवर्धनम् ।
आरोग्यं च पटुत्वं च करणानां प्रजायते ॥ 91

His body becomes extremely beautiful and his digestive fire increases. He does not fall ill and his faculties become sharp.

भूतार्थं च भविष्यं च वेत्ति सर्वस्य भाषणम् ।
अश्रुतान्यपि शास्त्राणि सरहस्यं वदेद् ध्रुवम् ॥ 92

He knows what has really happened and what is to happen in the future, and he understands the speech of everyone. He is certain to recite sacred texts which he hasn't even heard, together with their secret doctrines.

वक्त्रे सरस्वती देवी सदा नृत्यति निर्भरम् ।
मन्त्रसिद्धिर्भवेत्तस्य जपादेव न संशयः ॥ ९३

The goddess Sarasvati forever dances with abandon in his mouth. Through repetition he is sure to attain perfection of the mantra.

जरामरणदुःखौघान्नाशयति गुरोर्वचः ।
इदं ध्यानं सदा कार्यं पवनाभ्यासिना परम् ।
ध्यानमात्रेण योगीन्द्रो मुच्यते नात्र संशयः ॥ ९४

The word of the guru destroys old age, death, and a host of sorrows. This great meditation is to be performed regularly by the practitioner of pranayama. Merely through meditation the master yogi is sure to be freed from every sin.

मूलपद्मं यदा ध्यायेत्स्वयम्भूलिंगसंज्ञकम् ।
तदा तत्क्षणमात्रेण पापौघं नाशयेद् ध्रुवम् ॥ ९५

When the yogi meditates upon the Muladhara lotus, which is called the self-born linga, he is sure to destroy all his sins immediately.

यद्यत्काम्यते चित्ते तत्तत्फलमवाप्नुयात् ।
निरन्तरकृताभ्यासात्तं पश्यति विमुक्तिदम् ॥ ९६

He obtains whatever reward he desires in his mind. Through constant practice he sees the giver of liberation.

बाह्यादभ्यन्तरं श्रेष्ठं पूजनीयं प्रयत्नतः ।
तन्त्रे श्रेष्ठतमं ह्येतन्नान्यदस्ति मतं मम ॥ 97

The internal meditation is better than the external and
should be carefully cultivated. This is the very best meditation in the tantra. I approve of no other.

आत्मसंस्थं शिवं त्यक्त्वा बहिःस्थं यः समर्चयेत् ।
हस्तस्थं पिण्डमुत्सृज्य भ्रमते जीविताशया ॥ 98

He who rejects the internal Shiva and worships the
external casts aside the food in his hand to wander in
search of sustenance.

आत्मलिंगार्चनं कुर्यादिनालस्यो दिने दिने ।
तस्य स्यात्सकला सिद्धिर्नत्र कार्या विचारणा ॥ 99

Complete perfection arises for him who tirelessly worships
his internal linga every day. This is not to be doubted.

निरन्तरकृताभ्यासात्षण्मासैः सिद्धिमाप्नुयात् ।
तस्य वायुप्रवेशोऽपि सुषुम्णायां भवेद् ध्रुवम् ॥ 100

Through constant practice the yogi attains perfection
within six months. His breath is sure to enter Sushumna.

मनोजयं च लभते वायुबिन्दुविधारणम् ।
ऐहिकामुष्मिकी सिद्धिर्भवेन्नैवात्र संशयः ॥ 101

He conquers his mind, checks his breath and bindu, and attains perfection both in this world and the next. In this there is no doubt.

द्वितीयं च सरोजं यल्लिंगमूले व्यवस्थितम् ।
तद्‍ब्वादिलान्तषड्वर्णं परिभास्वरषड्दलम् ॥ 102

The second lotus, which is found at the base of the penis, contains six syllables,[8] starting with *ba* and ending in *la*, and has six shining petals.

स्वाधिष्ठानाभिधं तत्तु पंकजं शोणरूपकम् ।
बालाख्यो यत्र सिद्धोऽस्ति देवी यत्रास्ति राकिनी ॥ 103

That lotus is called Svadhishthana and is red. The adept called Bala and the goddess Rakini reside in it.

यो ध्यायति सदा नित्यं स्वाधिष्ठानारविन्दकम् ।
तस्य कामांगनाः सर्वा भजन्ते काममोहिताः ॥ 104

All beautiful women become besotted with and adore the man who regularly meditates upon the eternal Svadhishthana lotus.

विविधं चाश्रुतं शास्त्रं निःशंको वै वदेद् ध्रुवम् ।
सर्वरोगविनिर्मुक्तो लोके चरति निर्भयः ॥ 105

---

[8]The six syllables are *ba, bha, ma, ya, ra,* and *la.*

And he is sure to proclaim unhesitatingly various sacred texts that he has not heard before. Free from all disease, he wanders about the world fearlessly.

मरणं खाद्यते तेन स केनापि न खाद्यते ।
तस्य स्यात्परमा सिद्धिरणिमादिगुणप्रदा ॥ 106

He devours death and nothing devours him. He gets the ultimate perfection, which bestows the powers of becoming infinitesimal and so forth.

वायुः संचरते देहे रसवृद्धिर्भवेद् ध्रुवम् ।
आकाशपंकजगलत्पीयूषमपि वर्द्धते ॥ 107

Breath flows in his body and his fluids are sure to increase. The nectar flowing from the lotus in the ether also increases.

तृतीयं पंकजं नाभौ मणिपूरकसंज्ञकम् ।
दशारं डादिफान्तार्णं स्वर्णवर्णं सुशोभितम् ॥ 108

The third lotus is at the navel and is called Manipuraka. It has ten spokes, contains the syllables from *ḍa* to *pha*,[9] has the color gold, and is beautiful.

तत्र सिद्धो भुजंगाख्यो लाकिनी तत्र देवता ॥ 109

---

[9]The syllables are *ḍa, ḍha, ṇa, ta, tha, da, dha, na, pa,* and *pha.*

The adept there is called Bhujanga and the goddess
is Lakini.

तस्मिन्ध्यानं सदा योगी करोति मणिपूरके ।
तस्य पातालसिद्धिः स्यान्निरन्तरसुखावहा ॥ 110

When the yogi regularly meditates on Manipuraka, he
gets Patala siddhi,[10] the bringer of unceasing bliss.

ईप्सितं च भवेल्लोके दुःखरोगविनाशनम् ।
कालस्य वंचनं चापि परदेहप्रवेशनम् ॥ 111

He gets what he wants here in this world, he gets rid of
suffering and disease, he can cheat death, and he can
enter another's body.

जाम्बुनदादिकरणं सिद्धानां दर्शनं भवेत् ।
ओषधीदर्शनं चापि निधीनां दर्शनं तथा ॥ 112

He can create gold and suchlike, see the adepts, find
elixirs, and discover buried treasures.

हृदयेऽनाहतं नाम चतुर्थं पंकजं भवेत् ।
कादिठान्तार्णसंस्थानं द्वादशारसमन्वितम् ॥ 113

---

[10]Patala siddhi is the ability to journey to the underworlds.

In the heart is the fourth lotus, known as Anahata.
The syllables from *ka* to *ṭha*[11] are found there and it has
twelve spokes.

अतिशोणं कामराजप्रसादस्थानमीरितम् ।
पद्मस्थं तत्परं तेजो बाणलिंगं प्रकीर्तितम् ॥ 114

It is bright red and said to be the location of the palace
of Kamaraja. The great light in the lotus is called
the banalinga.[12]

तस्य स्मरणमात्रेण दृष्टादृष्टफलं भवेत् ।
सिद्धः पिनाकी यत्रास्ते काकिनी यत्र देवता ॥ 115

Merely by thinking of it, the reward of knowing one's
past and future lives arises. The adept there is Pinaki and
the goddess is Kakini.

एतस्मिन्सततं ध्यानं हृत्पाथोजे करोति यः ।
क्षुभ्यन्ते तस्य कान्या वै कामार्ता दिव्ययोषितः ॥ 116

When a man meditates constantly upon this lotus in
the heart, divine maidens are excited by his beauty and
fall in love.

---

[11]These syllables are *ka, kha, ga, gha, ṅa, ca, cha, ja, jha, ña, ṭa,* and *ṭha.*
[12]Banalinga is another name for a narmadeshvara, a stone found in the river
  Narmada and worshipped as a natural lingam.

ज्ञानं चाप्रतिमं तस्य त्रिकालविषयं भवेत् ।
दूरश्रुतिर्दूरदृष्टिः स्वेच्छया खगतां व्रजेत् ॥ 117

He gets a matchless knowledge of the past, present, and future, long-distance hearing and sight, and he can move through the air at will.

सिद्धानां दर्शनं चापि योगिनीदर्शनं तथा ।
भवेत्खेचरसिद्धिश्च खेचराणां जयं तथा ॥ 118

He can see adepts and yoginis, and he gets Khechara siddhi and mastery over the khecharas.[13]

यो ध्यायति परं नित्यं बाणलिंगं द्वितीयकम् ।
खेचरीभूचरीसिद्धिर्भवेत्तस्य न संशयः ॥ 119

He who regularly meditates on the second great banalinga is sure to get Khechari and Bhuchari siddhis.

एतद्ध्यानस्य माहात्म्यं कथितुं नैव शक्यते ।
ब्रह्माद्याः सकला देवा गोपयन्ति परं त्विदम् ॥ 120

The power of this great meditation is indescribable. Brahma and all the other gods keep it secret.

कण्ठस्थानस्थितं पद्मं विशुद्धं नाम पंचमम् ।

---

[13]A khechara is a divine being, literally one who moves (-chara) in the ether (khe-).

सुहेमाभं सुरोपेतं षोडशस्वरशोभितम् ॥ 121

The fifth lotus is in the throat and called Vishuddha. It is golden, contains gods, and is adorned with sixteen syllables.

छगलण्डोऽस्ति सिद्धोऽत्र शाकिनी चाधिदेवता ।
ध्यानं करोति यो नित्यं स योगीश्वरपण्डितः ॥ 122

The adept there is Chagalanda and the presiding goddess is Shakini. He who regularly meditates on it is a wise man amongst master yogis.

किं तस्य योगिनोऽन्यत्र विशुद्धाख्ये सरोरुहे ।
चतुर्वेदा विभासन्ते रहस्यानि विधेरिव ॥ 123

What need of anything else for the yogi who meditates on the Vishuddha lotus? The four Vedas become manifest in him, as do the secrets of fate.

इह स्थाने स्थितो योगी यदा क्रोधवशो भवेत् ।
तदा समस्तं त्रैलोक्यं कम्पते नात्र संशयः ॥ 124

When the yogi is meditating on that region and becomes angry, all the three worlds are sure to tremble.

इह स्थाने मनो यस्य दैवाद्याति लयं यदा ।
तदा बाह्यां परित्यज्य स्वान्तरे रमते चिरम् ॥ 125

When his mind happens to become absorbed in this place, the yogi rejects what is outside him and dwells happily within himself for a long time.

तस्य न क्षतिरायाति स्वशरीरस्य शक्तितः ।
संवत्सरसहस्रेऽपि वज्रातिकठिनस्य वै ॥ 126

Through its power, his body is harder than diamond and does not deteriorate even in a thousand years.

यदा त्यजति तद्ध्यानं योगीन्द्रोऽवनिमण्डले ।
तदा वर्षसहस्राणि मन्यते तत्क्षणं कृती ॥ 127

When the expert master yogi stops this meditation, he reckons thousands of years here on earth to be an instant.

आज्ञापद्मं भ्रुवोर्मध्ये हंक्षोपेतं द्विपत्रकम् ।
शुक्लाभं तन्महाकालः सिद्धो देव्यत्र हाकिनी ॥ 128

The Ajna lotus is between the eyebrows. It contains the syllables *ham* and *ksha* and has two petals. It is white, its adept is Mahakala, and the goddess there is Hakini.

शरच्चन्द्रनिभं तत्राक्षरबीजं विजृम्भितम् ।
पुमान्परमहंसोऽयं यज्ज्ञात्वा नावसीदति ॥ 129

A syllabic seed syllable is found there which looks like the autumn moon. The man who knows it is a paramahamsa and never perishes.

एतदेव परं तेजः सर्वतन्त्रेषु मन्त्रितम् ।
चिन्तयित्वा परां सिद्धिं लभते नात्र संशयः ॥ 130

This same great light is discussed in all the tantras.
By contemplating it, the yogi is sure to attain the
supreme perfection.

तुरीयं त्रितयं लिंगं तदहं मुक्तिदायकः ।
ध्यानमात्रेण योगीन्द्रो मत्समो भवति ध्रुवम् ॥ 131

That third linga is the highest mental state; it is I, the
giver of liberation. Merely by meditating on it, the master
yogi is sure to become like me.

इडा हि वरणाख्याता पिंगलासीति होच्यते ।
वाराणासी तयोर्मध्ये विश्वनाथोऽत्र भाषितः ॥ 132

Ida is called Varana, Pingala is called Asi. Between them
is Varanasi. Vishvanatha is said to be there.[14]

एतत्क्षेत्रस्य माहात्म्यमृषिभिस्तत्त्वदर्शिभिः ।
शास्त्रेषु बहुधा प्रोक्तं परं तत्त्वं सुभाषितम् ॥ 133

The importance of his domain has been declared many
times in the sacred texts by sages who know the ultimate
truth. It is well described as the Ultimate Reality.

---

[14]Varana and Asi are two rivers which join the Ganga, or Ganges, in Varanasi.
The most important temple to Shiva in Varanasi is that of Vishvanatha.

सुषुम्णा मेरुणा याता ब्रह्मरन्ध्रं यतोऽस्ति वै ।
ततश्चैषा परावृत्य तदाज्ञापद्मदक्षिणे ।
वामनासापुटं याति गंगेति परिगीयते ॥ 134

Sushumna goes by way of Meru to the aperture of
Brahman and comes back from there via the right side
of the Ajna lotus to the left nostril. She is celebrated
as Ganga.

ब्रह्मरन्ध्रे हि यत्पद्मं सहस्रारं व्यवस्थितम् ।
तत्र कन्दे हि या योनिस्तस्यां चन्द्रो व्यवस्थितः ॥ 135

The lotus situated in the aperture of Brahman is the
Sahasrara. In the bulb there is a yoni, in which is
situated the moon.

त्रिकोणाकारतस्तस्याः सुधा क्षरति निश्चितम् ।
इडायाममृतं तत्र समं स्रवति चन्द्रमाः ॥ 136

The yoni is triangular and nectar constantly flows from
it. The moon makes the nectar of immortality there flow
directly into Ida.

अमृतं तद्द्रहति सा धारारूपं निरन्तरम् ।
वामनासापुटं याति गंगेत्युक्ता हि योगिभिः ॥ 137

She constantly carries that nectar of immortality in the
form of a stream. She goes to the left nostril and is called
Ganga by yogis.

आज्ञापंकजदक्षांशाद्वामनासापुटं गता ।
उदग्वहैव तत्रेडा वरणा समुदाहृता ॥ 138

Ida goes from the right side of the Ajna lotus to the left
nostril. There she flows upwards and is called Varana.[15]

तदाकारा पिंगलापि तदाज्ञाकमलोत्तरे ।
दक्षनासापुटे याति प्रोक्तास्माभिरसीति वै ।
ततो द्वयमिह स्थाने वाराणस्यां तु चिन्तयेत् ॥ 139

Pingala has the same form on the left of the Ajna lotus.
It goes to the right nostril and I call it Asi. Thus one
should visualize those two in that place, which is
called Varanasi.

मूलाधारे हि यत्पद्मं चतुष्पत्रं व्यवस्थितम् ।
तत्र कन्देऽस्ति या योनिस्तस्यां सूर्यो व्यवस्थितः ॥ 140

In the bulb in the Muladhara, which is the lotus with four
petals, is a yoni, in which is situated the sun.

तत्सूर्यमण्डलाद्घोरं विषं क्षरति संततम् ।
पिंगलायां विषं तत्र समर्पयति तापनः ॥ 141

From the orb of the sun a terrible poison drips constantly.
The sun offers the poison to Pingala there.

---

[15]Udagvaha, which has been translated as "flows upwards" can also mean "flows
in the north." In Varanasi, the Varana is found on the north side of the city.

विषं तत्र वहन्ती या धारारूपं निरन्तरम् ।
दक्षनासापुटं याति कल्पितेयं तु पूर्ववत् ॥ 142

The channel which constantly conveys the poison there
in the form of a stream goes to the right nostril and is
fashioned like the one before.

आज्ञापंकजवामांशाद्दक्षनासापुटं गता ।
उद्ग्वहा पिंगलापि पुरासीति प्रकीर्तिता ॥ 143

Pingala also goes from the left side of the Ajna lotus to
the right nostril, flowing upwards. It was earlier said
to be called Asi.

आज्ञापद्ममिदं प्रोक्तं यत्र देवो महेश्वरः ।
पीठत्रयं ततश्चोर्ध्वं निरुक्तं योगचिन्तकैः ।
तद्विन्दुनादशक्त्याख्यं भालपद्दे व्यवस्थितम् ॥ 144

The place where the god Maheshvara is found is called
the Ajna lotus, and above that, those who know Yoga
have declared there to be a triad of sacred abodes,
namely bindu, nada, and shakti, situated on the surface
of the forehead.

यः करोति सदा ध्यानमाज्ञापद्दे तु गोपितम् ।
पूर्वजन्मकृतं कर्म स्मृतं स्यादविरोधतः ॥ 145

He who regularly practices the secret meditation on the
Ajna lotus will remember with ease what he has done
in former lives.

इह स्थितो यदा योगी ध्यानं कुर्यान्निरन्तरम् ।
तदा करोति प्रतिमां प्रति जल्पनमर्थवत् ॥ 146

When the resolute yogi meditates unceasingly upon it,
he holds a meaningful conversation with the image.

यक्षराक्षसगन्धर्वा अप्सरोगणकिन्नराः ।
सेवन्ते चरणौ तस्य सर्वे तस्य वशानुगाः ॥ 147

Yakshas, rakshasas, gandharvas, apsarases, ganas, and
kinnaras wait at his feet and are all under his control.

करोति रसनां योगी प्रविष्टां विपरीतगाम् ।
लम्बिकोर्ध्वेषु गर्तेषु धृत्वा ध्यानं भयापहम् ॥ 148

After practicing the meditation which dispels fear, the
yogi turns back his tongue and inserts it into the cavities
above the uvula.

अस्मिन्स्थाने मनो यस्य क्षणार्धं वर्ततेऽचलम् ।
तस्य सर्वाणि पापानि संक्षयं यान्ति तत्क्षणात् ॥ 149

All the sins of the yogi whose mind remains fixed on this
place for half an instant are instantly destroyed.

यानि यानीह प्रोक्तानि पंचपद्मे फलानि वै ।
तानि सर्वाणि सुतरामेतद्ध्यानाद्भवन्ति हि ॥ 150

By meditating on it all the rewards which have here
been said to be found in the first five lotuses arise to a
greater degree.

यः करोति सदाभ्यासमाज्ञापद्मे विचक्षणः ।
वासनाया महाबन्धं तिरस्कृत्य प्रमोदते ॥ 151

The wise man who regularly carries out the practice
on the Ajna lotus casts aside the great bondage of past
impressions and is blissful.

प्राणप्रयाणसमये तत्पदं यः स्मरत्सुधीः ।
त्यजेत्प्राणं स धर्मात्मा परमात्मनि लीयते ॥ 152

At the time of his lifebreath leaving, the wise and dutiful
man who is thinking of that lotus as he casts it off is
absorbed into the supreme self.

तिष्ठन्गच्छन्स्वपन्भुञ्जन्यो ध्यानं कुरुते नरः ।
पापकर्मापि कुर्वाणो न हि मज्जति किल्बिषे ॥ 153

The man who practices this meditation while sitting,
walking, sleeping, and eating, does not sink into sin even
if he performs bad acts.

राजयोगाधिकारी स्यादेतच्चिन्तनतो ध्रुवम् ।
योगी द्वन्द्वविनिर्मुक्तः स्वीयया प्रभया स्वयम् ॥ 154

Through meditating on this, the yogi is sure to earn the right to practice Raja Yoga and be freed from dualities by means of his own personal splendor.

द्विदलध्यानमाहात्म्यं कथितुं नैव शक्यते ।
ब्रह्मादिदेवताश्चैव किंचिन्मत्तो विदन्ति ते ॥ 155

The importance of meditation on the lotus with two petals cannot be put into words. Even Brahma and the other gods learn a little of it from me.

अत ऊर्ध्वं तालुमूले सहस्रारं सरोरुहम् ।
अस्ति यत्र सुषुम्णाया मूलं सविवरं स्थितम् ॥ 156

Above it, at the root of the palate, is the Sahasrara[16] lotus, in which is situated the opening where the Sushumna starts.

तालुमूले सुषुम्णा सा अधोवक्त्रा प्रवर्तते ।
मूलाधारेण योन्यन्ताः सर्वनाडीः समाश्रिताः ।
ता बीजभूतातीवतन्वी ब्रह्ममार्गप्रदायिकाः ॥ 157

At the root of the palate is Sushumna. She faces downwards. All nadis go via the Muladhara and end at

---

[16]Sahasrara literally means "thousand-spoked," i.e., "thousand-petaled."

the yoni. They are born of seed syllables, are extremely delicate, and show the way to Brahman.

तालुस्थाने च यत्पद्मं सहस्रारं पुरोदितम् ।
तत्कन्दे योनिरेकास्ति पश्चिमाभिमुखी मता ॥ 158

In the bulb of the lotus at the root of the palate, which has already been taught to be the Sahasrara, there is understood to be a single backwards-facing yoni.

तस्या मध्ये सुषुम्णाया मूलं सविवरं स्थितम् ।
ब्रह्मरन्ध्रं तदेवोक्तमामूलाधारपंकजम् ।
तत्तन्तुरन्ध्रे तच्छक्तिः प्रसुप्ता कुण्डली सदा ॥ 159

In its middle is situated the opening where the Sushumna starts. That is called the aperture of Brahman and goes as far as the Muladhara lotus, in the aperture of whose fine stem its shakti, Kundalini, is constantly sleeping.

सुषुम्णायां स्थिता नाडी चित्रा स्यान्मम वल्लभा ।
तस्यां मम मते कार्या ब्रह्मरन्ध्रादिकल्पना ॥ 160

In the Sushumna is found the Chitra nadi, which is dear to me. In my doctrine, the aperture of Brahman and so forth are to be conceived of as being situated in her.

यस्याः स्मरणमात्रेण सर्वज्ञत्वं प्रजायते ।
पापक्षयश्च भवति न भूयः पुरुषो भवेत् ॥ 161

Merely by thinking of her, omniscience arises, sins are destroyed, and the yogi is never again born as a man.

प्रवेशितं स्वलांगूलं मुखे स्वस्य निवेशयेत् ।
तेनात्र न वहत्येव देहचारी समीरणः ॥ 162

The yogi should insert her tail into her mouth and keep it there. As a result, the wind that moves in the body completely ceases to flow there.

तेन संसारचक्रेऽस्मिन्न भ्रमत्येव सर्वदा ।
तदर्थं वै प्रवर्तन्ते योगिनः प्राणधारणे ॥ 163

Consequently, the yogi does not go around forever on this wheel of samsara. That is why yogis practice breath retention.

तत एवाखिला नाड्यो निरुद्धाश्चाष्टवेष्टना ।
इयं कुण्डलिनी शक्ती रन्ध्रं त्यजति नान्यथा ॥ 164

Only as a result of this—and not otherwise—are all the nadis closed off, and does this Kundalini shakti, with her eight coverings, leave the opening.

यदा पूर्णासु नाडीषु संनिरुद्धोऽनिलस्तदा ।
बन्धत्यागेन कुण्डल्या मुखं रन्ध्राद्बहिर्भवेत् ॥ 165

When the breath in all the nadis is restrained, then, as a result of shaking off its shackles, the mouth of Kundalini emerges from the opening.

सुषुम्णायां सदैवायं वहेत्प्राणसमीरणः ।
मूलपद्मस्थिता योनिर्वामदक्षिणकोणतः ॥ 166

The prana breath always flows in Sushumna. The yoni is situated with its left and right corners at the root lotus.

इडापिंगलयोर्मध्ये सुषुम्णा योनिमध्यगा ।
ब्रह्मरन्ध्रं तु तत्रैव सुषुम्णाधारमण्डले ।
यो जानाति स मुक्तः स्यात्कर्मबन्धाद्विचक्षणः ॥ 167

The Sushumna is between Ida and Pingala, in the middle of the yoni, and the aperture of Brahman is right there, in the region of the base of the Sushumna. The wise man who knows this is freed from the bondage of karma.

ब्रह्मरन्ध्रमुखे तासां संगमः स्यादसंशयः ।
यस्मिन्स्नाते स्नातकानां मुक्तिः स्याद्विरोधतः ॥ 168

The confluence of these three is without doubt at the mouth of the aperture of Brahman. Those who bathe in it are sure to get liberation.

गंगायमुनयोर्मध्ये वहत्येषा सरस्वती ।
तासां तु संगमे स्नात्वा धन्यो याति परां गतिम् ॥ 169

It is Sarasvati who flows in the middle of Ganga and Yamuna. The lucky man who bathes in their confluence goes to the ultimate destination.

इडा गंगा पुरा प्रोक्ता पिंगला चार्कपुत्रिका ।
मध्या सरस्वती ज्ञेया तासां संगोऽतिदुर्लभः ॥ 170

Ida has already been said to be Ganga, and Pingala the daughter of the sun.[17] The one in the middle is said to be Sarasvati. Their confluence is extremely hard to find.

सितासिते संगमे यो मनसा स्नानमाचरेत् ।
सर्वपापविनिर्मुक्को याति ब्रह्म सनातनम् ॥ 171

He who mentally bathes in the white and black confluence[18] is freed from all sins and goes to the eternal Brahman.

त्रिवेण्यां संगमे यो वै पितृकर्म समाचरेत् ।
तारयित्वा पितृन्सर्वान्स याति परमां गतिम् ॥ 172

He who performs ancestor rituals at the Triveni confluence[19] brings about salvation for all his ancestors and goes to the ultimate destination.

---

[17]"Daughter of the sun" is another name for the Yamuna river.

[18]The waters of the Yamuna have a dark hue; those of the Ganga are light.

[19]Triveni means "having three braids" and is the name of the confluence of the Ganga and Yamuna (and Sarasvati) at Prayag, modern-day Allahabad.

नित्यं नैमित्तिकं काम्यं प्रत्यहं यः समाचरेत् ।
मनसा चिन्तयित्वा तु सोऽक्षयं फलमाप्नुयात् ॥ 173

He who mentally performs the obligatory, occasional, and
optional rites every day obtains an everlasting reward.

सकृद्यः कुरुते स्नानं स्वर्गे सौख्यं भुनक्ति सः ।
दग्ध्वा पापानशेषान्वै योगी शुद्धमतिः स्वयम् ॥ 174

The pure-minded yogi who bathes in it once, automatically burns up all his sins and enjoys pleasure in heaven.

अपवित्रः पवित्रो वा सर्वावस्थां गतोऽपि वा ।
स्नानाचरणमात्रेण पूतः भवति नान्यथा ॥ 175

Impure, pure, or in any condition, merely by bathing in it
he becomes purified, and not otherwise.

मृत्युकाले पुतं देहं त्रिवेण्याः सलिले यदा ।
विचिन्त्य यस्त्यजेत्प्राणं स सदा मोक्षमाप्नुयात् ॥ 176

At the time of death, the man who imagines his body
bathed in the waters of Triveni before casting off his lifebreath always obtains liberation.

नातः परतरं गुह्यं त्रिषु लोकेषु विद्यते ।
गोप्तव्यं तत्प्रयत्नेन न चाख्येयं कदाचन ॥ 177

No greater secret than this is to be found in the three worlds. It is to be guarded carefully and never told.

ब्रह्मरन्ध्रे मनो दत्त्वा क्षणार्धं यदि तिष्ठति ।
सर्वपापविनिर्मुक्तः स याति परमां गतिम् ॥ 178

If a man puts his mind at the aperture of Brahman and remains there for half an instant, he is freed from all sins and goes to the ultimate destination.

अस्मिंल्लीनं मनो यस्य स योगी मयि लीयते ।
अणिमादिगुणान्भुक्त्वा स्वेच्छया पुरुषोत्तमः ॥ 179

The yogi whose mind is absorbed in it is absorbed in me. That finest of men freely enjoys the powers of becoming infinitesimal and so forth.

एतद्रन्ध्रध्यानमात्रेण मर्त्यः संसारेऽस्मिन्वल्लभो मे भवेत्सः ।
पापं जित्वा मुक्तिमार्गाधिकारी ज्ञानं दत्त्वा तारयाम्याशु तं वै ॥ 180

Merely by meditating on this aperture a man here in the world of samsara overcomes sin, becomes dear to me, and earns the right to journey on the path to liberation. I shall give him knowledge and quickly make him cross to the other side.

चतुर्मुखादित्रिदशैरगम्यं योगिवल्लभम् ।
प्रयत्नेन सुगोप्यं तद्ब्रह्मरन्ध्रं मयोदितम् ॥ 181

This aperture of Brahman of which I have spoken is inaccessible to four-faced Brahma and the other gods, dear to yogis, and to be carefully kept secret.

पुरा मयोक्ता या योनिः सहस्रारे सरोरुहे ।
तस्याधो वर्तते चन्द्रस्तद्ध्यानं क्रियते बुधैः ॥ 182

Below the yoni, in the Sahasrara lotus, which has already been described by me, is the moon. The wise practice meditation on it.

यस्य स्मरणमात्रेण योगीन्द्रोऽवनिमण्डले ।
पूज्यो भवति देवानां सिद्धानां सम्मतो भवेत् ॥ 183

Merely by thinking of it, the lord of yogis becomes worthy here on earth of worship by the gods, and is held in esteem by the adepts.

शिरःकपालविवरे ध्यायेद्दुग्धमहोदधिम् ।
तत्र स्थित्वा सहस्रारे पद्मे चन्द्रं विचिन्तयेत् ॥ 184

The yogi should visualize an ocean of milk in the space in the skull. Remaining there, he should imagine the moon in the Sahasrara lotus.

शिरःकपालविवरे द्विरष्टकलया युतः ।
पीयूषभानुर्हंसाख्यस्तारयेत्तं निरञ्जनम् ॥ 185

It is in the space in the skull, has sixteen digits, is known as the moonswan, has rays made of nectar, and will make the pure yogi cross to the other side.

निरन्तरकृताभ्यासात्त्रिदिनैः पश्यति ध्रुवम् ।
दृष्टिमात्रेण पापौघं दहत्येव स साधकः ॥ 186

Through constant practice, within three days the aspirant is sure to have a revelation and, merely by that vision, he burns up a mass of sins.

अनागतं च स्फुरति चित्तशुद्धिर्भवित्खलु ।
सद्यः कृत्वापि दहति महापातकपंचकम् ॥ 187

As soon as he does so, the future becomes manifest, his mind is purified, and he burns up the five great sins.[20]

आनुकूल्यं ग्रहा यान्ति सर्वे नश्यन्त्युपद्रवाः ।
उपसर्गाः शमं यान्ति युद्धे जयमवाप्नुयात् ॥ 188

The planets become favorable, all disasters are no more, problems cease, and he is victorious in battle.

खेचरीभूचरीसिद्धिर्भवित्क्षीरेन्दुदर्शनात् ।
ध्यानादेव भवेत्सर्वं नात्र कार्या विचारणा ॥ 189

---

[20]The five sins are killing a Brahmin, drinking alcohol, stealing, sleeping with one's guru's wife, and associating with anyone guilty of these crimes.

From seeing the moon in the milk, Khechari and Bhuchari siddhis arise. Through visualization alone all this arises. This is not to be doubted.

सतताभ्यासयोगेन सिद्धो भवति मानवः ।
सत्यं सत्यं पुनः सत्यं मम तुल्यो भवेद् ध्रुवम् ।
योगशास्त्रेऽप्यभिरतं योगिनां सिद्धिदायकम् ॥ 190

Through constant application of the practice a man becomes perfected. Truly, truly, and again truly, the yogi is sure to become equal to me. That which is cherished in the texts of Yoga bestows perfection upon yogis.

अत ऊर्ध्वं दिव्यरूपं सहस्रारं सरोरुहम् ।
ब्रह्माण्डाख्यस्य देहस्य बाह्ये तिष्ठति मुक्तिदम् ॥ 191

Above there, outside the body which is called the egg of Brahma, is the divinely beautiful Sahasrara lotus which bestows liberation.

कैलासो नाम तस्यैव महेशो यत्र विद्यते ।
अकुलाख्योऽविनाशी च क्षयवृद्धिविवर्जितः ॥ 192

It is called Kailasa, and Mahesha lives there under the name Akula. He is imperishable, free from decay or growth.

स्थानस्यास्य ज्ञानमात्रेण नृणां संसारेऽस्मिन्संभवो नैव भूयः ।

भूतग्रामं संतताभ्यासयोगात्कर्तुं हर्तुं स्याच्च शक्तिः समग्रा ॥ 193

Just by knowing this place, men are not born again here in samsara. Through regular application of the practice, the power to create and destroy all living beings arises in its entirety.

स्थाने परे हंसनिवासभूते कैलासनाम्नीह निविष्टचेताः ।
योगी हतव्याधिरधःकृताधिबाधश्चिरं जीवति मृत्युमुक्तः ॥ 194

With his mind fixed on this great place, which is the abode of the swan and is called Kailasa, the yogi is freed from disease, casts off illness and affliction, and lives for a long time, liberated from death.

चित्तवृत्तिर्यदा लीनाकुलाख्ये परमेश्वरे ।
तदा समाधिसंपन्नो योगी निश्चलतां व्रजेत् ॥ 195

When the operation of the mind is focused on Para-meshvara, under the name of Akula, then the yogi has perfected samadhi and becomes unchanging.

निरन्तरकृताद्ध्यानाज्जगद्विस्मरणं भवेत् ।
तदा विचित्रसामर्थ्यं योगिनो भवति ध्रुवम् ॥ 196

When the yogi practices the meditation constantly, he becomes oblivious to the world, and then he is sure to get various wonderful powers.

अस्मान्गलितपीयूषं पिबेद्योगी निरन्तरम् ।
मृत्युमृत्युं विधायाशु कुलं जित्वा सरोरुहम् ॥ 197

Having brought about the death of death and quickly
overcome the Kula lotus, the yogi should constantly
drink the nectar which drips from there.

अत्र कुण्डलिनी शक्तिर्लयं याति कुलाभिधा ।
तदा चतुर्विधा सृष्टिर्लीयते परमात्मनि ॥ 198

Here Kundalini shakti, which is called Kula, obtains
absorption. Then the fourfold creation is absorbed into
the supreme self.

यन्नत्वा प्राप्य विषयं चित्तवृत्तिर्विलीयते ।
तस्मिन्परिश्रमं योगी करोति निरपेक्षकः ॥ 199

On reaching there, the operations of the mind find an
object and become absorbed. The disinterested yogi
strives for this.

चित्तवृत्तिर्यदा लीना तस्मिन्योगी भवेद् ध्रुवम् ।
तदा विजयतेऽखण्डज्ञानरूपि निरञ्जनम् ॥ 200

When the operations of the mind are absorbed in the
object, one assuredly becomes a yogi. Then the pure
essence, which has the form of unbroken knowledge,
is triumphant.

ब्रह्माण्डबाह्ये संचिन्त्य स्वप्रतीकं यथोदितम् ।
तमावेश्य महच्छून्यं चिन्तयेद्विरोधतः ॥ 201

The yogi should visualize his own image outside the egg of Brahma as described previously, insert it into the great void, and meditate freely upon it.

आद्यन्तमध्यशून्यं तत्कोटिसूर्यसमप्रभम् ।
चन्द्रकोटिप्रतीकाशमभ्यस्य सिद्धिमाप्नुयात् ॥ 202

It has no beginning, middle, or end, is as bright as ten million suns, and has the splendor of ten million moons. After carrying out the practice on it, the yogi attains success.

एतद्ध्यानं सदा कुर्यादिनालस्यो दिने दिने ।
तस्य स्यात्सकला सिद्धिर्वत्सरान्नात्र संशयः ॥ 203

He should practice this meditation tirelessly every day. After a year he will get complete success. In this there is no doubt.

क्षणार्धं निश्चलं तत्र मनो यस्य भवेद् ध्रुवम् ।
तस्य कल्मषसंघातस्तत्क्षणादेव नश्यति ॥ 204

All the sins of he whose mind is fixed there without moving for half a moment are instantly destroyed.

यं दृष्ट्वा न निवर्तते मृत्युसंसारवर्त्मनि ।
अभ्यसेत्तं प्रयत्नेन स्वाधिष्ठानेन वर्त्मना ॥ 205

After seeing it, the yogi does not meet his end on the road of death and transmigration. He should zealously carry out that practice via the path of the Svadhishthana.

एतद्ध्यानस्य माहात्म्यं मया वक्तुं न शक्यते ।
यः साधयति जानाति सोऽस्माकमपि संमतः ॥ 206

I cannot explain the importance of this meditation. He who masters it understands and is held in respect by me.

ध्यानादेव विजानाति विचित्रं क्षणसंभवम् ।
अणिमादिगुणोपेतो भवत्येव न संशयः ॥ 207

Only through meditation does the yogi recognize the various things that arise momentarily and is he sure to obtain the powers of becoming infinitesimal and so forth.

राजयोगो मयाख्यातः सर्वतन्त्रेषु गोपितः ।
राजाधिराजयोगं हि कथयामि समासतः ॥ 208

I have taught the Raja Yoga which is concealed in all the tantras. Now I shall teach in brief the Rajadhiraja Yoga.[21]

---

[21]Raja Yoga literally means "King Yoga," i.e., the king of Yogas, and Rajadhiraja Yoga is the "king of kings" amongst Yogas.

स्वस्तिकं चासनं कृत्वा सुमठे जन्तुवर्जिते ।
गुरुं संपूज्य यत्नेन ध्यानमेतत्समाचरेत् ॥ 209

In a pleasant hermitage where there are no other living
beings, the yogi should assume Svastikasana, carefully
worship his guru, and practice this meditation.

निरालम्बो भवेज्जीवो ज्ञात्वा वेदान्तयुक्तितः ।
निरालम्बं मनः कृत्वा न किंचिच्चिन्तयेत्सुधीः ॥ 210

After obtaining knowledge through the reasoning of
Vedanta, the jiva becomes freestanding. The wise man
should make his mind freestanding and not think
of anything.

एतद्ध्यानान्महासिद्धिर्भवत्येव न संशयः ।
वृत्तिहीनं मनः कृत्वा पूर्णरूपः स्वयं भवेत् ॥ 211

Great success is sure to arise as a result of this meditation. Having made the mind free of fluctuations, the yogi
automatically becomes complete.

साधयेत्सततं यो वै स योगी विगतस्पृहः ।
अहं नाम न कोऽप्यस्मिन्सर्वदात्मैव विद्यते ॥ 212

The yogi who practices constantly becomes desireless.
There is no 'I.' At all times, only the self exists in him.

को बन्धः कस्य वा मोक्ष एकं पश्येत्सदा हि सः ।
एतत्करोति यो नित्यं स मुक्तो नात्र संशयः ।
स एव योगी मद्भक्तः सर्वलोकेषु पूजितः ॥ 213

What is bondage? Who is liberated? The yogi always sees
unity. He who does this continually is liberated. In this
there is no doubt. He alone is a yogi, devoted to me, worshipped in all the worlds.

अहमस्मीति च यदा जीवात्मपरमात्मनोः ।
अहंतदेतदुभयं त्यक्त्वाखण्डं विचिन्तयेत् ॥ 214

When the yogi identifies himself with the individual and
supreme selves he should abandon the pair 'I' and 'that'
and meditate on that which is undivided.

अध्यारोपापवादाभ्यां यत्र सर्वं विलीयते ।
तद्बीजमाश्रयेद्योगी सर्वसंगविवर्जितः ॥ 215

Free from all attachment, the yogi should take refuge
in that seed in which all things vanish by means of
realizing that they have been incorrectly understood
and dismissing them.

अपरोक्षं चिदानन्दं पूर्णं त्यक्त्वा भ्रमाकुलाः ।
परोक्षमपरोक्षं च कृत्वा मूढा भ्रमन्ति वै ॥ 216

Having cast aside that which is knowable, complete consciousness, and bliss, those confused by misunderstanding

make the unknowable the knowable, and wander about
at a loss.

चराचरमिदं विश्वं परोक्षं यः करोति च ।
अपरोक्षं परं ब्रह्म त्यक्त्वा तस्मिन्प्रलीयते ॥ 217

One who acts on this movable and immovable universe,
which is unknowable—and casts aside the supreme
Brahman, which is knowable—he is absorbed in
the unknowable.

ज्ञानकारणजं ज्ञानं यथा नोत्पद्यते भृशम् ।
अभ्यासं कुरुते योगी तथा संगविवर्जितः ॥ 218

In order that knowledge produced by the organs of
knowledge does not arise excessively, the yogi should
carry out the practice free from attachment.

सर्वेन्द्रियाणि संयम्य विषयेभ्यो विचक्षणाः ।
सुषुप्ता इव तिष्ठन्ति सर्वसंगविवर्जिताः ॥ 219

Restraining their senses from all objects of the senses,
wise men live as if in deep sleep, free from all attachment.

एवमभ्यसतो नित्यं स्वप्रकाशः प्रकाशते ।
श्रोतुर्बुद्धौ समप्यार्थं निवर्तन्ते गुरोर्गिरः ।
तदभ्यासवशादेकं स्वतो ज्ञानं प्रवर्तते ॥ 220

An inner illumination shines forth from the yogi who regularly practices thus. The guru's words yield their meaning in the mind of the listener and then exist no more. Through the power of this practice, a unique knowledge develops automatically.

यतो वाचो निवर्तन्ते अप्राप्य मनसा सह ।
साधनादमलं ज्ञानं स्वयं स्फुरति तद् ध्रुवम् ॥ 221

Through application of the practice, that pure knowledge is sure to shine forth automatically, from which words, in the company of the mind, turn back, having been unable to reach it.

हठं विना राजयोगो राजयोगं विना हठः ।
न सिध्यति ततो युग्ममानिष्पत्तेः समभ्यसेत् ।
तस्मात्प्रवर्तते योगी हठे सद्गुरुमार्गतः ॥ 222

Without Hatha, Raja Yoga does not succeed, nor does Hatha succeed without Raja Yoga. So the yogi should practice both until they are complete. Hence he undertakes Hatha following the path of a good guru.

स्थिते देहे जीवति यो अधुना न म्रियते भृशम् ।
इन्द्रियार्थोपभोगेषु स जीवति न संशयः ॥ 223

He who does not now quickly die in his body while it is unchanging and alive, lives for the enjoyment of the objects of the senses. In this there is no doubt.

अभ्यासपाकपर्यन्तं मितान्नशरणो भवेत् ।
अन्यथा साधनं धीमान्कर्तुं पारयतीह न ॥ 224

Until the practice is complete, the yogi should resort to a restricted diet. Without doing so, a wise man is unable to carry out the practice in this life.

अतीव साधुसंलापं त्यजेत्संसदि बुद्धिमान् ।
करोति पिण्डरक्षार्थं बह्वालापविवर्जितः ॥ 225

The clever man should not talk too much with the good men in the assembly. He should do enough to take care of his person, avoiding excessive chatter.

त्यजतां त्यजतां संगं सर्वथा त्यजतां भृशम् ।
अन्यथा न लभेन्मुक्तिं सत्यं सत्यं मयोदितम् ॥ 226

The yogi must, but must, abandon company. He has to do it completely and utterly, otherwise he will not get liberation. Truly, I have spoken the truth.

गृहे वै क्रियतेऽभ्यासः संगं त्यक्त्वा तदन्तरे ।
व्यवहाराय कर्तव्यो बाह्ये संगो न रागतः ॥ 227

The practice is to be performed indoors at home, shunning company. Company is to be kept outdoors for the sake of everyday business, without attachment.

स्वे स्वे कर्मणि वर्तन्ते सर्वे ते कर्मसंभवाः ।
निमित्तमात्रकरणे न दोषोऽस्ति कदाचन ॥ 228

All those who are the products of action are busy with their own particular actions. There is never anything wrong with an action whose cause is only occasional.

एवं निश्चित्य सुधिया गृहस्थोऽपि यदाचरेत् ।
तदा सिद्धिमवाप्नोति नात्र कार्या विचारणा ॥ 229

He who realizes this and conducts himself intelligently is sure to obtain perfection, even if he is a householder.

पापपुण्यविनिर्मुक्तः परित्यक्तांगसंगकः ।
यो भवेत्स विमुक्तः स्याद्गृहे तिष्ठन्सदा गृही ॥ 230

He who is free from sin and merit and has foregone bodily contact is liberated, even if he always lives in a house as a householder.

पापपुण्यैर्न लिप्येत योगयुक्तो सदा गृही ।
कुर्वन्नपि च पापानि स्वकार्ये लोकसंग्रहे ॥ 231

The householder who constantly applies himself to Yoga does not incur sin or merit, even if he performs sinful deeds when carrying out his duties for the good of the world.

अधुना संप्रवक्ष्यामि मन्त्रसाधनमुत्तमम् ।
ऐहिकामुष्मिकसुखं येन स्यादविरोधतः ॥ 232

Now I shall teach the best mantra practice, by means of
which the pleasures of this world and the next are sure
to arise.

यस्मिन्मन्त्रवरे ज्ञाते योगसिद्धिर्भवेत्खलु ।
योगिनः साधकेन्द्रस्य सर्वैश्वर्यसुखप्रदा ॥ 233

When this best of mantras is known, success in Yoga,
which bestows absolute dominion and pleasure, will
indeed arise for the yogi who is the best of practitioners.

मूलाधारेऽस्ति यत्पद्मं चतुर्दलसमन्वितम् ।
तन्मध्ये वाग्भवं बीजं विस्फुरन्तं तडित्प्रभम् ॥ 234

In the middle of the lotus with four petals in the
Muladhara is the Vagbhava seed syllable, flashing like a
bolt of lightning.

हृदये कामराजं तु बन्धूककुसुमप्रभम् ।
आज्ञारविन्दे शक्त्याख्यं चन्द्रकोटिसमप्रभम् ॥ 235

In the heart is the Kamaraja, which looks like a bandhuka
flower. In the Ajna lotus is the seed syllable called Shakti
which looks like ten million moons.

बीजत्रयमिदं गोप्यं भुक्तिमुक्तिफलप्रदम् ।
एतन्मन्त्रत्रयं योगी साधयेत्सिद्धिसाधकः ॥ 236

This triad of seed syllables grants the rewards of both
worldly enjoyment and liberation. The yogi striving to
achieve perfection should master these three mantras.

एतन्मन्त्रं गुरोर्लब्ध्वा न द्रुतं न विलम्बितम् ।
अक्षराक्षरसन्तानं निःसंदिग्धमना जपेत् ॥ 237

After receiving this mantra from his guru, the yogi
should repeat all of its syllables in sequence, neither
quickly nor slowly, his mind free from doubt.

तन्नतश्रैकचित्तश्च शास्त्रोक्तविधिना सुधीः ।
देव्यास्तु पुरतो लक्षं हुत्वा लक्षत्रयं जपेत् ॥ 238

Absorbed in it, his mind one-pointed, the wise yogi
should make one lakh oblations before the goddess in the
manner described in the sacred texts and then repeat the
mantra three lakh times.

करवीरप्रसूनं तु गुडक्षीरराज्यसंयुतम् ।
कुण्डे योन्याकृतौ धीमान् जपान्ते जुहुयात्सुधीः ॥ 239

At the end of the repetition, the wise and clever yogi
should offer an oblation of oleander blossom mixed with
jaggery, milk, and ghee into a fire pit in the shape of a yoni.

अनुष्ठाने कृते ह्यस्मिन्पूर्वसेवाकृता भवेत् ।
ततो ददाति कामान्वै देवी त्रिपुरभैरवी ॥ 240

When this observance has been performed, the goddess
Tripurabhairavi, created by the earlier worship, appears
and grants wishes.

गुरुं संतोष्य विधिवल्लब्ध्वा मन्त्रवरं त्विमम् ।
अनेन विधिना युक्तो मन्दभाग्योऽपि सिध्यति ॥ 241

Having duly pleased his guru and obtained this finest
of mantras, even an unlucky yogi can achieve success by
means of this technique.

लक्षमेकं जपेद्यस्तु साधको विजितेन्द्रियः ।
दर्शनात्तस्य क्षुभ्यन्ते योषितो मदनातुराः ।
पतन्ति साधकस्याग्रे निर्लज्जा भयवर्जिताः ॥ 242

At the sight of the practitioner who repeats it one lakh
times with his senses subdued, women tremble and
become sick with love. They fall shameless and without
fear before the practitioner.

जप्तेन च द्विलक्षेण ये यस्मिन्विषये स्थिताः ।
आगच्छन्ति यथा तीर्थं विमुक्तकुलविग्रहाः ।
ददते तस्य सर्वस्वं तस्यैव च वशे स्थिताः ॥ 243

Repeated two lakh times, it makes men living in the
region come as if to a place of pilgrimage, abandoning

their families and possessions. They give him all their property and are under his power.

त्रिभिर्लक्षैस्तथा जप्तैर्माण्डलिकाः समण्डलाः ।
वशमायान्ति ते सर्वे नात्र कार्या विचारणा ।
षड्भिर्लक्षैर्महीपालः सभृत्यबलवाहनः ॥ 244

And when it is repeated three lakh times, all the district governors are sure to be subjugated, together with their districts. With six lakh repetitions, the king is subjugated, together with his dependents, his troops, and his vehicles.

लक्षैर्द्वादिशकैर्जप्तैर्यक्षरक्षोरगेश्वराः ।
वशमायान्ति ते सर्वे आज्ञां कुर्वन्ति नित्यशः ॥ 245

With twelve lakh repetitions, yakshas, rakshasas, and great snakes all come under his control and do his bidding forever.

त्रिपंचलक्षैर्जप्तैस्तु साधकेन्द्रस्य धीमतः ।
सिद्धविद्याधराश्चैव सगन्धर्वाप्सरोगणाः ॥ 246
वशमायान्ति ते सर्वे नात्र कार्या विचारणा ।
दूरश्रवणविज्ञानं सर्वज्ञत्वं प्रजायते ॥ 247

When it is repeated fifteen lakh times, adepts and sorcerers, together with gandharvas, apsarases, and ganas, are sure to come under the control of the wise master practitioner. Long-distance hearing, clairvoyance, and omniscience arise.

तथाष्टादशभिर्लक्षैर्देहिनानेन साधकः ।
उत्तिष्ठेन्मेदिनीं त्यक्त्वा दिव्यदेहस्तु जायते ।
भ्रमते स्वेच्छया लोकेऽछिद्रां पश्यति मेदिनीम् ॥ 248

And with eighteen lakh repetitions, using this body the practitioner leaves the ground and rises up. He gets a divine body, wanders freely about the universe, and sees the earth in its perfect entirety.

अष्टाविंशतिभिर्लक्षैर्विद्याधरपतिर्भवेत् ।
साधकस्तु भवेद्धीमान्कामरूपो महाबलः ॥ 249

With twenty-eight lakh repetitions, the practitioner becomes the lord of the sorcerers, wise, able to assume any form he wishes, and very powerful.

त्रिंशल्लक्षैस्तथा जपैर्ब्रह्मविष्णुसमो भवेत् ।
रुद्रत्वं षष्टिभिर्लक्षैः शक्तितत्त्वमशीतिभिः ॥ 250

And with thirty lakh repetitions, he becomes equal to Brahma and Vishnu. With sixty lakh, he attains the state of Rudra. With eighty, he becomes the principle of Shakti.

कोट्यैकया महायोगी लीयते परमे पदे ।
साधकस्तु भवेद्योगी त्रैलोक्ये सोऽतिदुर्लभः ॥ 251

With one crore repetitions, the great yogi is absorbed into the Absolute. The practitioner becomes a yogi of great rarity in the three worlds.

त्रिपुरे त्रिपुरं त्वेकं शिवं परमकारणम् ।
अक्षयं तत्पदं शान्तमप्रमेयमनामयम् ।
लभतेऽसौ न सन्देहो धीमान्सर्वमभीप्सितम् ॥ 252

O Tripura! That wise man is sure to obtain the one Shiva Tripura, the supreme cause, that imperishable, peaceful, immeasurable, healthy abode—everything that is desired.

शिवविद्या महाविद्या गुप्ता चाग्रे महेश्वरि ।
मद्भाषितमिदं शास्त्रं गोपनीयमतो बुधैः ॥ 253

Shiva's magical science is a great magical science and has been kept secret from the outset, O Great Goddess. Therefore, this treatise that I have spoken should be kept secret by the wise.

हठविद्या परं गोप्या योगिना सिद्धिमिच्छता ।
भवेद्वीर्यवती गुप्ता निर्वीर्या च प्रकाशिता ॥ 254

The magical science of Hatha is to be very well guarded by the yogi desirous of success. Guarded, it becomes powerful; made public, it becomes powerless.

य इदं पठते नित्यमाद्योपान्तं विचक्षणः ।

योगसिद्धिर्भवेत्तस्य क्रमेणैव न संशयः ॥ 255

The wise man who regularly reads this treatise from beginning to end is sure gradually to obtain success in Yoga.

स मोक्षं लभते धीमान्य इदं नित्यमर्चयेत् ।
मोक्षार्थिभ्यश्च सर्वेभ्यः साधुभ्यः श्रावयेदपि ॥ 256

The wise man who regularly worships this treatise
obtains liberation, and he should recite it to all good men
who seek liberation.

क्रियायुक्तस्य सिद्धिः स्यादक्रियस्य कथं भवेत् ।
तस्मात्क्रिया विधानेन कर्तव्या योगिपुंगवैः ॥ 257

Success arises for he who is intent upon the practice. How
can it arise for he who does not practice? Thus the finest
yogis should carry out the practice according to the rules.

यदृच्छालाभसंतुष्टः संत्यक्तान्तरसंगकः ।
गृहस्थः स कृताशेषो मुक्तः स्याद्योगसाधनैः ॥ 258

The householder who is content with whatever he
happens to obtain, who has given up inner attachment,
and who has completed all the practices becomes liberated
by means of the techniques of Yoga.

गृहस्थानां भवेत्सिद्धिरीश्वराराधनेन वै ।

योगक्रियाभियुक्तानां तस्मात्संयतते गृही ॥ 259

Householders intent on the practice of Yoga achieve perfection through worshiping the Lord, so a householder should engage himself in the struggle.

गेहे स्थिता पुत्रदारादिपूर्णे संगं त्यक्त्वा चान्तरे योगमार्गे ।
सिद्धेर्श्रिहं वीक्ष्य पश्चाद्गृहस्थः क्रीडेत्सो वै मे मतं साधयित्वा ॥ 260

Living in a house filled with children and a wife and so forth, internally abandoning attachment, and then seeing the mark of success on the path of Yoga, the householder has fun having mastered my teaching."

इति श्रीशिवसंहितायां योगशास्त्रे ईश्वरपार्वतीसंवादे
पंचमः पटलः ॥

Thus ends the fifth chapter in the glorious *Shiva Samhita*, a treatise on Yoga in the form of a dialogue between the Lord and Parvati.

Contributors

JAMES MALLINSON is a graduate of Eton and Oxford, holds a master's from the School of Oriental and African Studies, University of London, and returned to Oxford University for his doctorate. He has also spent years in India, living amongst the yogis.

SHIPRA, the woman in the photographs, is by profession a physiotherapist and by avocation a yogini and a model. She lights up the runways in New Delhi.
MUNISH KHANNA is one of India's most versatile and innovative photographers. Trained in New York and based in New Delhi, his work has appeared in leading publications worldwide. You can find out more at MunishKhanna.com.

YOGAVIDYA.COM is dedicated to publishing excellent and affordable books about Yoga. It is completely independent of any commercial, governmental, educational, or religious institutions.

Index

Page numbers in *italics* refer to photographs.